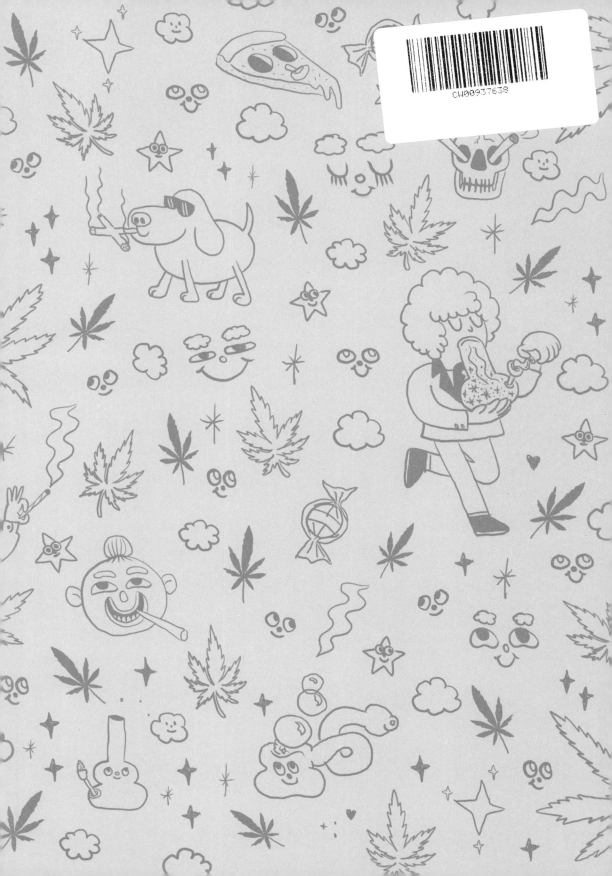

CW00937638

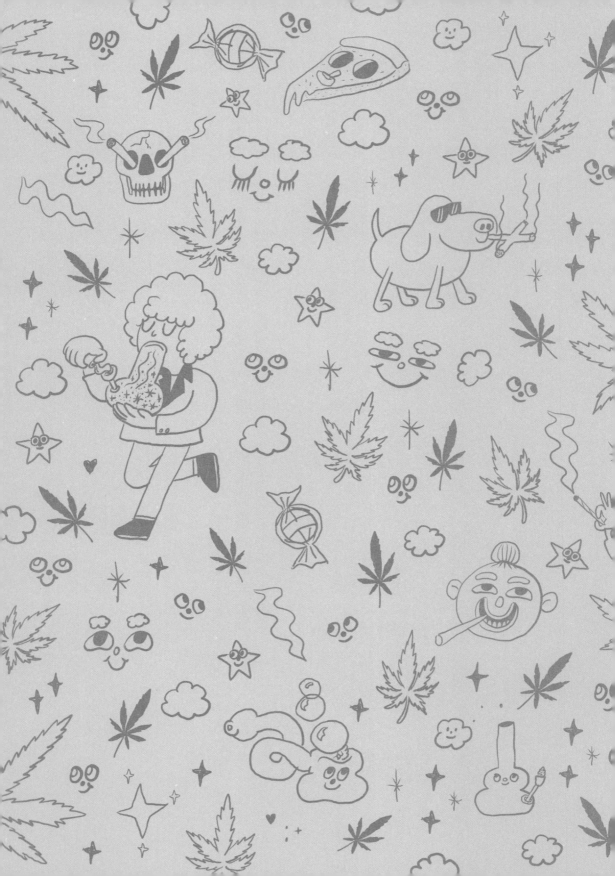

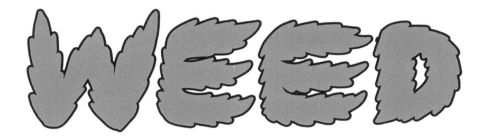

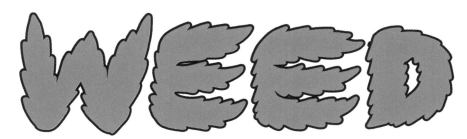

WEED

EVERYTHING YOU WANT TO KNOW BUT ARE ALWAYS TOO STONED TO ASK

MICHELLE LHOOQ

ILLUSTRATED BY

THU TRAN

PRESTEL

MUNICH · LONDON · NEW YORK

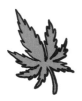
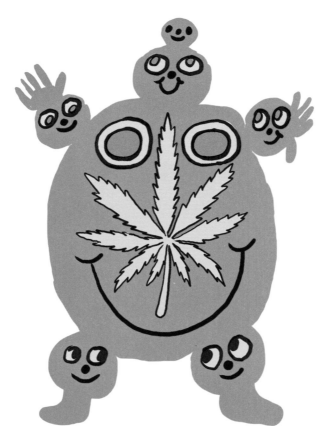

CONTENTS

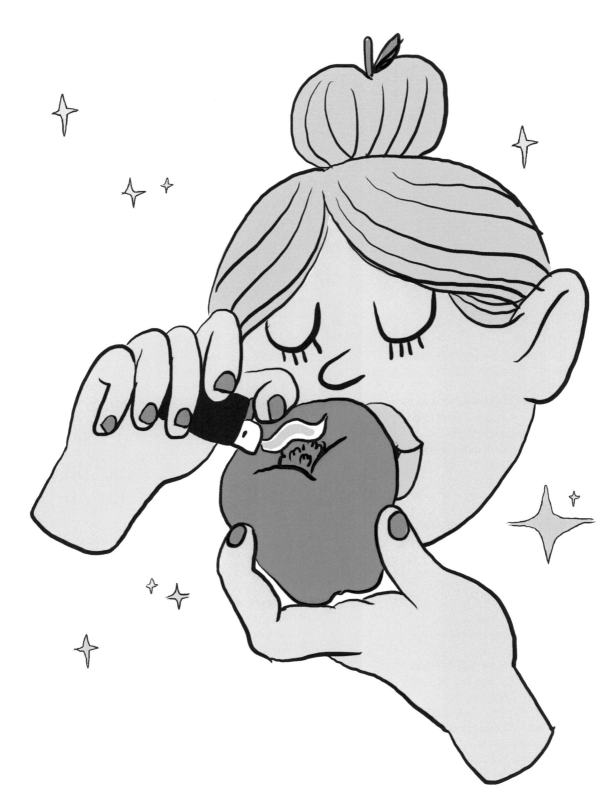

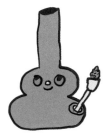

INTRODUCTION:
HOW DID WE GET HERE?

WEED! Maybe you've always been curious. Maybe you just smoked your first joint. Or maybe, if you're like millions of other potheads, you've vowed to stay high till you die. Whatever it is, the age of legal cannabis has finally arrived. What a time to be alive.

In 2017 I moved from New York to Los Angeles, the new cannabis capital of the world (sorry, Amsterdam!). I'd spent most of my twenties as a music journalist for *VICE*, chasing raves all across the globe. Now, I wanted to witness the weed revolution.

Diving into the cannabis industry, I found myself at a lot of weird weed parties—from CBD sound baths headlined by Icelandic indie bands, to Hollywood mansions where models were hired to roll blunts by the pool while Snoop Dogg DJed in the living room. Looking around, I realized that weed culture is changing fast.

These days, we don't just hit a bong, drive to White Castle for a burger, then pass out. We vape, we dab, we microdose … we even *lube*. We put THC in our coffee, CBD in our soap, and juice cannabis leaves into smoothies. We go to

school to be budtenders, and spend spring break at cannabis resorts. Instead of tie-dye shirts, we lounge around in pot leaf streetwear. Instead of saying, "Dude … I'm stoned," we say, "I'm medicated."

I wanted to write about modern stoner culture and all its crazy developments. While there are many other pot manuals out there, this one is a roadmap to the new weed order, drawing on the cast of colorful characters I've met in the industry, as well as the stoner culture I've absorbed at nightclubs, raves, and festivals.

Coming up, you'll learn how to have high sex, bake vegan edibles, and find the coolest stoner hangouts in the world. You'll get pro tips from experts including a weed sommelier, a renegade farmer, and an iconic musician. Of course, some things never change, like how to roll the perfect joint and the proper way to pass it around a circle. We'll go over all of that too.

So if you've just started smoking weed, welcome to the party! You're late, but don't sweat it. The cops just showed up and said everything's cool. Now it's about to get *really* crazy.

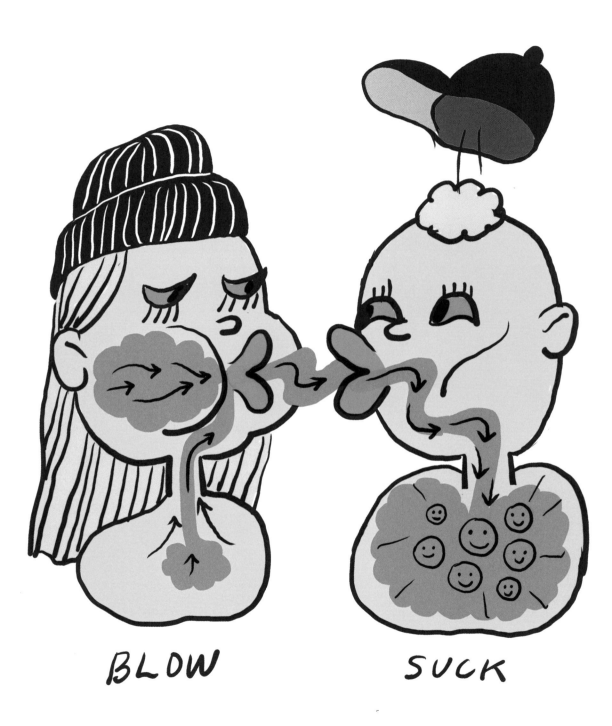

BLOW   SUCK

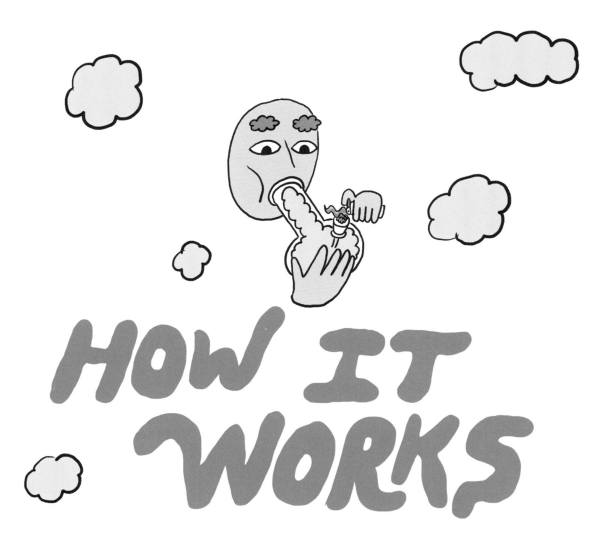

HOW IT WORKS

You know how, when you start at a new school or job, they always make you do some lame orientation activity? You wish you could skip it to get stoned instead, but you drag your butt through it anyway—and end up learning a bunch of stuff that, admittedly, it would have been more annoying to figure out on your own later.

This part of the book is Weed 101. Before we get into the smoking and cooking and love-making

(you knew this would get a little dirty…), we're starting with the basics: how the cannabis plant works from shoot to stem. Along the way, we'll dip into some advanced stoner stuff like cannabinoids and terpenes; you'll also get a crash course from a professional weed sommelier (*yes that is a real thing*) on how to train your nose.

Basically, this is where we'll try to open our eyes and see weed for what it is—and what it can be.

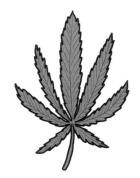

ANATOMY OF
A CANNABIS PLANT

Weed comes from the plant *Cannabis sativa* L., which likely originated in high-elevation areas of Central Asia, arriving in the tropics later. The plant flourishes in the wild, especially in warm climates—there's a reason it's called "weed," after all. While there are thousands of different cannabis strains, C. *sativa* L. can be divided into three subspecies: *sativa*, *indica*, and *ruderalis*. Here's a quick breakdown of what a cannabis plant looks like:

Flowers (AKA "Buds")
The gloriously dank flowers of a female cannabis plant are what we're here for: this is what we call weed. As the wise sage Rihanna once said, "Baby, this is what you came for."

Resin (AKA "Kief")
The sticky layer of crystals covering the flowers of a mature plant are made up of microscopic, globe-like trichomes—potent little piñatas where compounds like THC and CBD are stored.

Seeds
We use these to grow plants. Seeds can be male or female, and while both plants produce flowers, only the female flowers are psychoactive—and they're therefore more valuable.

Sugar Leaves
Smaller leaves in the bud that contain some THC. They are typically trimmed out and used to make hash and edibles.

Fan Leaves
The big leaves that have become the universal symbol of weed.

Stalk/Stems
Cannabis stalks contain very little THC. When cannabis plants are bred for industrial purposes (hemp), their stalks can be used to make things like paper and textiles.

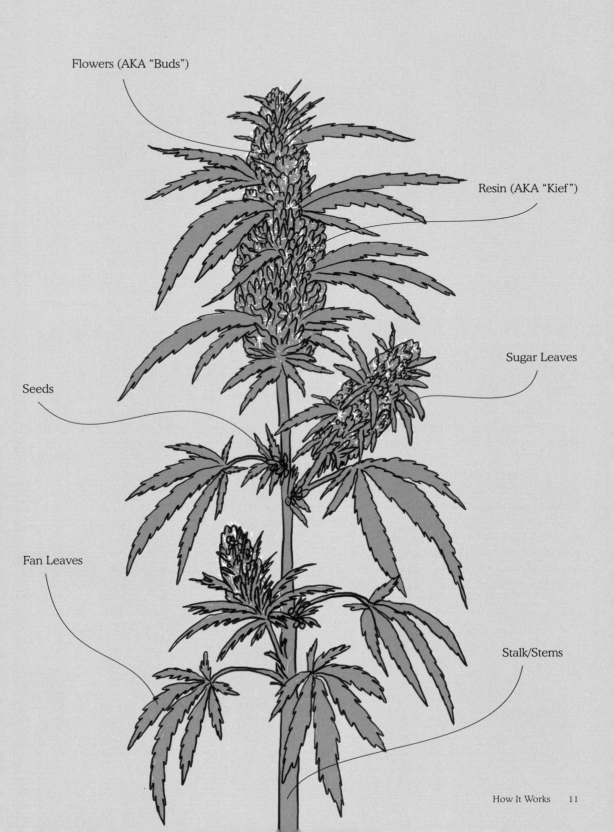

Flowers (AKA "Buds")

Resin (AKA "Kief")

Sugar Leaves

Seeds

Fan Leaves

Stalk/Stems

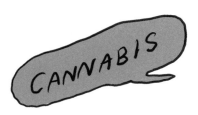

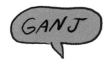

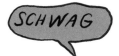

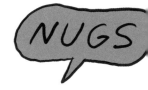

STONER SLANG

While almost everyone I know says "weed," there are hundreds of different ways to refer to cannabis, and the words we choose to use say a lot about society's evolving relationship to this plant.

The official term is "**cannabis**," which derives directly from the plant's scientific name. "Cannabis" comes from the Greek *kannabis* and means "hemp" in Latin. "**Marijuana**" is also a popular term and is believed to have come from the Mexican Spanish *marihuana*.

In recent years there has been a concerted push within the scientific and medical community to use "cannabis" as the standard, because of the troubling history of how "marijuana" came to be. In the 1930s, Harry J. Anslinger, head of the newly formed Federal Bureau of Narcotics, started using the word *marihuana* in his campaign to regulate the plant. Using this term purposely distanced the plant from its medical and industrial uses in order to place a disproportionate emphasis on its use among Mexican immigrants. The

government's villainization of weed over the next few decades continued along these racist lines, with "marihuana" painted as an evil drug used by criminals, entertainers, and other so-called lowlifes. Jazz musicians like Billie Holiday were famously hounded into ruin for their love of smoking what some called the "**Devil's lettuce**."

"**Pot**" also has Mexican Spanish roots—it comes from a drink called *potación de guaya* that blends weed with wine or brandy. The term first gained popularity during Prohibition in the 1920s and '30s and is most commonly used by smokers of the hippie generation. Hippies are also probably the only people who still say "**reefer**," another word with Mexican Spanish roots, coming from the Mexican slang term for a stoned person, *grifo*.

"**Kush**" can be a confusing one because it's commonly used as a blanket term for high-quality weed ("that's some dank kush, man"), but it actually refers to cannabis plants grown in the Hindu

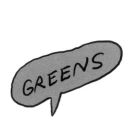

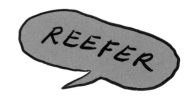

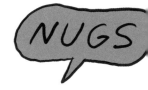

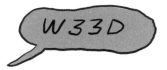

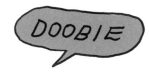

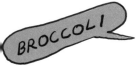

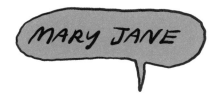

Kush region, on the border between Afghanistan and Pakistan.

On the other hand, no one will doubt what you're talking about when you say "**ganja**," which derives from the Sanskrit word for the hemp plant and is one of the oldest words for weed. (Although in my opinion, no one should use this term except for Rastafarians and New Age guru-types.)

There's also "**420**" ("four-twenty"), which was coined in the 1970s by five California high-schoolers after the time of day they would meet to smoke. Those three numbers are now synonymous with stoner culture, and led to April 20 being designated as the unofficial weed holiday. A bevy of other terms, like "**greens**," "**herb**," "**broccoli**," and "**tree**," are particularly useful when you're trying to be low-key.

And then there are hundreds more terms for the act of smoking weed, like "**taking a hit**," "**toking**," "**burning one**," and "**smoking up**."

"**Shotgunning**" is the act of inhaling smoke and blowing it into someone else's mouth—a commonly used (and sometimes creepy) make-out tactic. "**Smoking someone out**" means you're providing that person with free weed, while "**bogarting**" means you're committing the ultimate stoner foul: hogging the greens.

Getting really, really stoned—"**blazed**" or "**ripped**"—will give you "**cottonmouth**," an uncomfortable dry-mouth feeling, unless you're smoking "**schwag**," a commonly used term for low-quality weed. A "**roach**" is what you call the very end of a joint, while a "**crutch**" refers to the filter. If you're smoking a bong or pipe, "**it's cashed**" is how you let your friends know that someone needs to put more weed into the bowl.

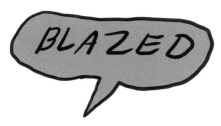

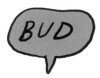

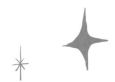

WHAT'S IN A STRAIN?

Whether or not strain names like "Jack Herer" and "OG Kush" really matter when it comes to predicting the kinds of effects weed will have is up for debate. "You know that dealers just make stuff up and put whatever will sell on the label, right?" a stoner friend once told me—a conspiracy theory, but one not completely beyond the realm of possibility.

Talking to a salesperson in a dispensary (or a stoner who likes to show off) can also be kind of intimidating. A typical conversation goes like this:

Budtender: Greetings, today we've got some top-shelf Blue Dream, a sativa-dominant hybrid that gives you full-body relaxation from the Blueberry indica, crossed with the buzzy, cerebral high of the Haze sativa. It's got a very nice blueberry aroma. We also have specials on the Bubba Kush, a pure and pungent indica akin to the Hindu Kush landrace strains, and AK-47, a hybrid with high THC content.

You: Um … they all sound pretty sweet … I'll take whatever you recommend?

But there's no need to get overwhelmed. Here are the facts: Cannabis typically comes in two main types, sativa and indica, and individual plants can be cross-bred to create an infinite variety of hybrids. Sativa flowers are long and narrow, and are associated with buzzy, electric highs. Indica flowers are short and squat, and induce more sedative, chill effects. Their resin is used to make hash.

Most strains these days are hybrids, so it's usually more accurate to say "sativa-dominant" or "indica-dominant"—with a note of caution, as some recent studies found that there was a very weak correlation between whatever sativa/indica percentage split it was claimed the plants had, and their actual genetic makeup. And while we usually assume that shared strain names like "Hindu Kush" and "Mango Kush" will have similar effects, studies suggest that might be a myth, too.

Nevertheless, the weed industry is moving toward strain specialization, with various cannabis awards and festivals feeding a market for celebrity, boutique, and exotic strains. New types are being bred every year, and, fascinatingly, many cannabis companies are moving away from traditional strain names and are instead labeling their pot after desired effects, like "Awake" or "Relaxed."

Regardless of which side you're on when it comes to the strain debate, there's no denying that weed is an incredibly multifaceted plant that can produce all kinds of different effects. Depending on your own body chemistry and what kind of cannabis you're smoking, you might feel energized or sluggish; buzzy or relaxed; super-social or super-shy. Sometimes it can cure your nausea—at other times it might make you even more sick. All of which is to say that if you come across a strain that really works for you, stick with it. Maybe it's your weed soulmate.

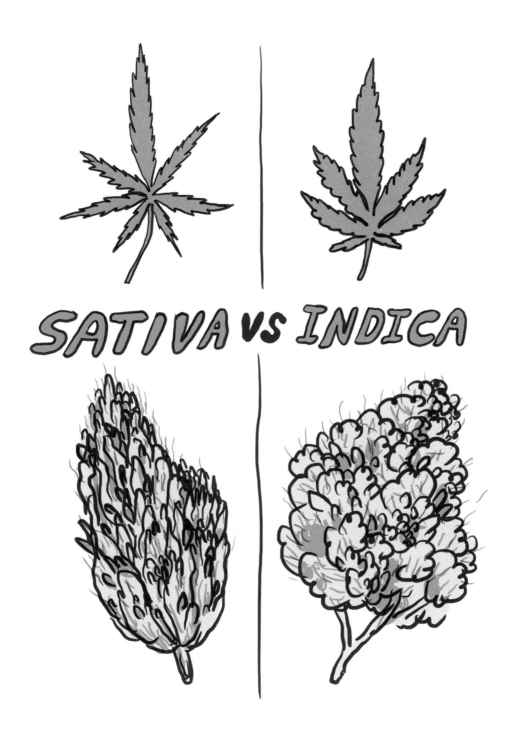

SATIVA vs INDICA

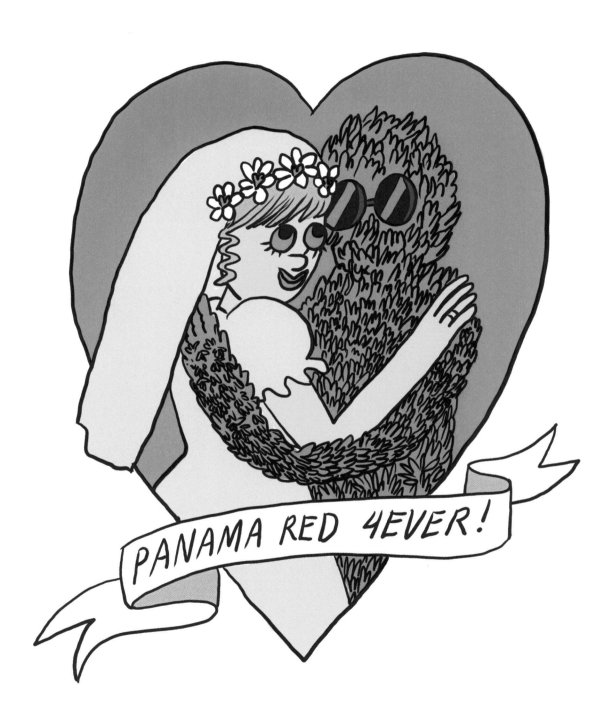

Weed Soulmates

I have a 100 percent accurate theory that everyone has a weed soulmate: one strain that works perfectly with your chemistry and makes you feel exactly the way you like.

Late one night on New York's Lower East Side, I was standing outside a music venue by myself when Actress, an experimental electronic musician from the UK, walked out. Actress is known for being kinda mysterious—in the show he'd just performed, he'd used a mannequin as a stand-in onstage while he DJed in the shadows. But when I floated this theory of weed soulmates to him, his face brightened up. "Oh yeah, mine's Blue Dream," he said, referring to an increasingly famous and popular sativa-dominant strain—the Kim Kardashian of weed strains, you could say.

A few months later, I decided to turn this idea into a column for *Merry Jane*, the weed website owned by Snoop Dogg. The first musician I interviewed was J-Cush, a London-by-way-of-New York DJ who runs a record label called Lit City Trax and literally named himself after weed. Appropriately, his weed soulmate is a type of very powerful kush—an indica-dominant hybrid called Private Reserve OG that's called the "Mike Tyson of strains" for its tendency to knock you out with one hit.

"I can only figure out if I love a certain kind of bud—if it agrees with me on a deeper level—after I've smoked a lot of it," J-Cush told me. He continued: "You might gel with someone straight away and want to spend more time together. But it's very hard to know if they're your soulmate off one encounter."

So screw the science. As a stoned Shakespeare might have said: *What's in a strain? That which we call weed, by any other word would smell as sweet.*

Popular Strains

Sativas	Indicas	Hybrids
Durban Poison	Afghani	Blue Dream
Green Crack	Blue Cheese	Cheese
Jack Herer	Blueberry	Girl Scout Cookies
Lemon Haze	Bubba Kush	Gorilla Glue
Panama Red	Kosher Kush	Headband
Purple Haze	Northern Lights	LA Confidential
Sour Diesel	OG Kush	NYC Diesel
Super Silver Haze	Pineapple Kush	Pineapple Express

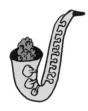

CANNABINOIDS

If you want to sound like a pro pothead, "cannabinoids," a group of chemical compounds found in cannabis, is the first term you're going to have to get familiar with. It's a bit of a tongue twister, but trust me, the instant stoner cred you'll get by dropping it in a conversation is so worth it.

Think of the cannabis plant like a giant orchestra. The instruments are coming together to create an overall impact while also each doing their own thing; sometimes working harmoniously, at other times contrasting or even counteracting one another. (At least, that's what I imagine— I haven't been to see an orchestra since I was a kid, if I'm totally honest.) Cannabinoids are like these instruments. They each have their own psychoactive or physical effects, but also combine to create what is called the "entourage effect." There are over eighty-five known cannabinoids in weed (some put the number closer to a hundred), but since research is still pretty limited, we are going to focus on the two major ones, THC and CBD, along with some rising contenders that are increasingly getting more attention, like CBN and THCA.

The reason why weed works so well with our bodies is thanks to our natural endocannabinoid system. Cannabis receptors were first discovered in the human body in 1988 by Dr. Allyn Howlett and her graduate student William Devane. There are two types of cannabinoid receptors in the human body. CB_1, found in the brain and nervous system, is involved in regulating processes like memory, cognition, pain sensation, and even our perception of time. CB_2 receptors, on the other hand, are mostly located in the nervous and immune systems, and work to reduce inflammation throughout the body. CB_2 receptors are even found in our skin, which is how cannabis lotions and salves work their soothing magic.

While these receptors interact with the body's natural endocannabinoids—like anandamide, which gives you that euphoric feeling after you've hit the gym—they also work with THC and other cannabinoids. So in a way, our bodies are made for weed.

Both governments and pharmaceutical companies around the world are looking to cash in on the benefits of cannabis by creating synthetic cannabinoids. This has resulted in medications that mimic the effects of weed, like Syndros, which was recently approved, and Marinol, which has been prescribed since the 1980s.

Since a lot of flower strains and concentrates, like THCA crystals (more on that later), are tailored these days to specific cannabinoids, it's definitely useful to know what you're getting yourself into the next time you're analyzing the label of a weed jar. "Ah yes, the cannabinoid content of these nugs is pure fire," you'll say to your impressed friend. Just kidding. Never say that.

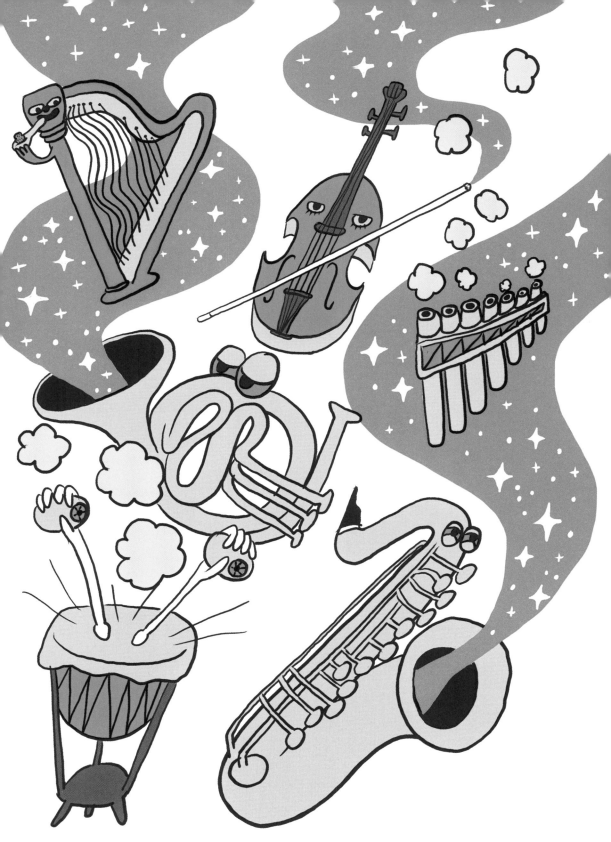

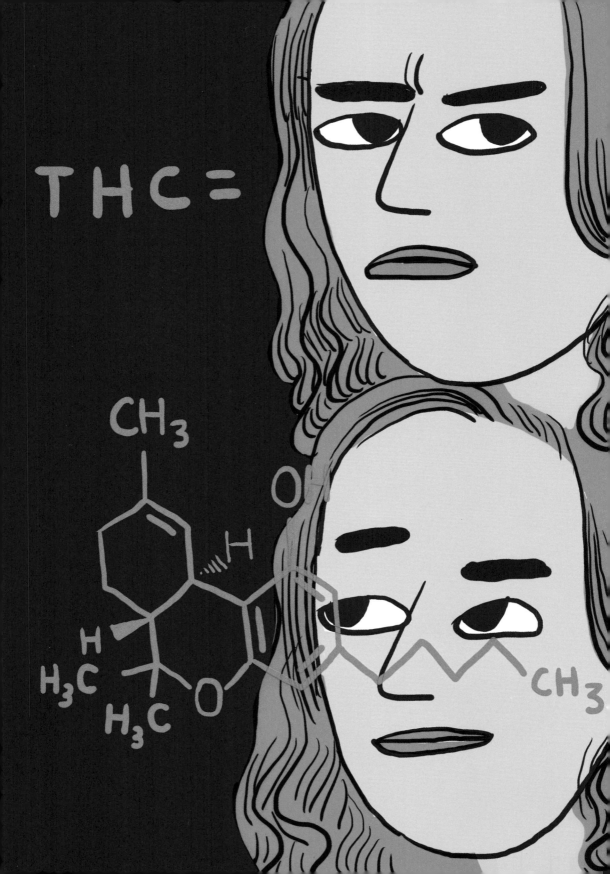

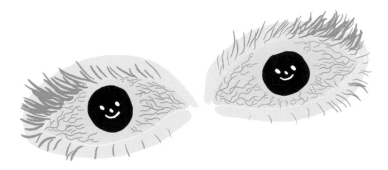

The Notorious THC

The cannabis plant contains hundreds of different chemical elements. But, for decades, everyone has been obsessed with just one of them: THC, or tetrahydrocannabinol, the most abundant (and notorious) cannabinoid in weed. THC was discovered by a Bulgarian-born Israeli chemist named Raphael Mechoulam. In 1964, he isolated and synthesized THC from Lebanese hashish, leading some to call him the "father of cannabinoid research." (Interesting side note: Israel has since become a leader in this field.)

This bad boy is what gets you stoned. It's psychoactive, stimulating your brain to perceive the world a little differently and start asking some hard-hitting questions (high thought: if tomatoes are a fruit, is tomato ketchup a smoothie?!). The THC "high" is really complex and variable. It can make you feel euphoric, relaxed, anxious, energetic, or stupid, depending on all kinds of factors like the type of strain, how your body chemistry reacts to it, and your own personal preferences. It's not all subjective, though—high levels of THC can increase the risk of paranoia and anxiety. Weed is also a lot more potent now than when the hippies were smoking it back in the day.

After decades of careful cultivation and improved technology, today's flower strains often hit around 20 percent THC, compared to less than 10 percent in the 1970s. Thankfully, in recent years growers have also started paying more attention to other cannabinoids, like CBD, which can counter the negative side-effects of getting too high.

THC might have some fascinating effects on the brain that we don't fully understand yet, too. Studies suggest that anandamide, an endocannabinoid known as the "bliss molecule" and which is sort of the human body's natural version of THC, may have something to do with the brain's ability to forget. This could be why THC has shown promise in clinical trials for treating trauma-related disorders like PTSD.

Finally, since it affects our bodies and immune systems, THC also has a ton of medical uses. It's a potent anti-inflammatory and can also relieve nausea, chronic pain, and digestive disorders like Crohn's disease. Certain strains, especially indicas, are particularly good at easing anxiety and relaxing your body so that you can drift off into a sweet, deep sleep.

An Old Stoner's Remedy

We've all been there. You're hanging out with your friends, hitting the L one more time even though you know you really shouldn't, or accidentally eating the whole weed brownie before someone says you were supposed to share. Suddenly you're sweating like rapper Trinidad James after popping a molly, your chest feels like a collapsible tent, and you're fighting the urge to call your mom (not that you could remember her number right now anyway—you've forgotten your own name). What do you do?

According to celebrated stoner Neil Young: chew some peppercorns. In October 2014, Young was a guest on Howard Stern's radio show, and the two were swapping stories when they landed on the topic of weed. "I do it every once in a while," Young told Stern, who replied that he stopped many years ago because he gets too paranoid. "Try black pepper balls," Young said. "Just chew two or three pieces. I just found this out myself. Try it."

Using black pepper to mellow out a too-intense high is an old stoner trick that actually dates all the way back to the Romans. It is mentioned in the ancient scholar Pliny the Elder's *Natural History*, from the first century CE, where he writes: "The gelotophyllis [literally 'leaves of laughter', or cannabis] grows in Bactria and along the Borysthenes. If this be taken in myrrh and wine all kinds of phantoms beset the mind, causing laughter which persists until the kernels of pine-nuts are taken with pepper and honey in palm wine."

Several scientific reviews in more recent years have also lent some credence to this theory, which is based on the fact that pepper contains beta-caryophyllene, a type of terpene (see p. 28) that

binds to the same cannabinoid receptors as THC but produces a counteractive, calming reaction. So the next time you find yourself spiraling on the verge of a weed freakout, grind up some fresh pepper and stick your nose in it like you're Kate Moss visiting Pete Doherty's recording studio. Take a big breath in. Sneeze. Immediately feel better.

THC Dosage Guide (for Smoking Buds)

Less than 8% = "I don't think this is working …"
8 to 16% = "I feel pretty great!"
16 to 25% = "I'm baked"
25% or higher = "I can read minds"

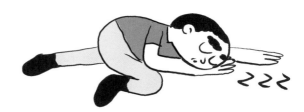

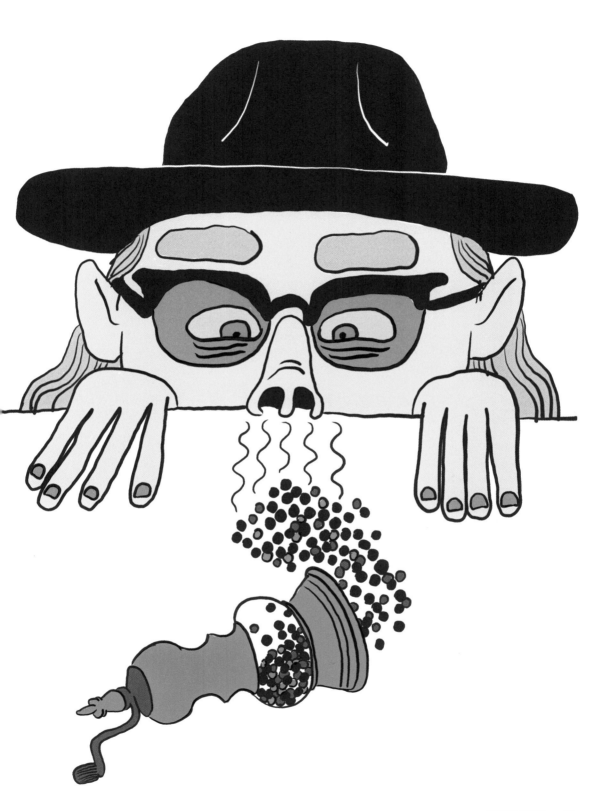

CBD, a Love Story

CBD, or cannabidiol, is the second most abundant chemical compound in weed after THC, and it can help to combat anxiety, inflammation, and pain. Research done over the last ten years suggests that CBD can also be used to treat a wide range of medical conditions; for example, cancer patients are given both THC and CBD to help with a range of ailments, including chemotherapy-induced nausea.

For the past few decades, cannabis plants have been bred to produce high levels of THC, a side effect being that levels of other cannabinoids in those plants has declined. Thus, CBD has been hidden in the shadow of its flashier, more popular older sister. THC and CBD are like Paris and Nicky Hilton—one is notorious for its limitless capacity for fun, while the other is more low-key and responsible, but just as cool in its own way.

Now that we're starting to understand the plant better, CBD is having a resurgence. You can even find it spiked in smoothies at music festivals and stocked in little bottles at the local natural foods store. It's non-psychoactive, which means you won't actually get "stoned"—useful when you're in a situation where you need to think straight. Basically, it's the perfect thing to take when you want to relax and feel better, like if you have really bad period cramps at school, or just want to go to bed. It's also ideal for people who don't usually smoke weed because they think it makes them super-paranoid. In fact, a 2006 study found that CBD actually counteracts the effects of THC, so it's a useful remedy if you accidentally get too stoned.

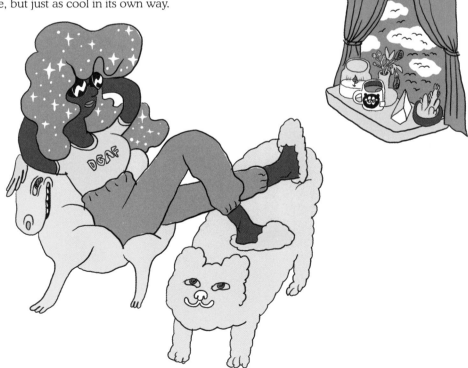

So You Want to Get Into CBD

Think of anything you can put in your mouth or on your body, and there is probably a CBD-infused version of it sold somewhere on the internet. While CBD exists in a legal gray zone in most countries, it's sold online and at health food stores all over the world. Even Amazon has gotten in on the action, so you really don't need to worry about cops busting down your door for ordering some CBD shampoo (seriously, that exists). Here's how to figure out the best product for you:

If you're about that vape life
CBD vapes are definitely the way to go. The Select brand's disposable CBD vapes are great because you don't have to worry about charging them up with a USB port. They come in delicious flavors like cinnamon, lavender, and grapefruit. CBD vapes are also one of the fastest ways to feel good.

If you want a good massage
Muscle-soothing CBD balms and lotions guarantee a next-level rubdown. Look for the ones infused with herbs like eucalyptus and peppermint for that full spa experience and satisfying tingly feeling. Apothecanna's creams are highly recommended as the stoner masseuse's go-to.

If you need quick pain relief
CBD tinctures and pills are the medical-grade solution for body ailments like aches and nausea. If you don't like puffing on vapes, popping these down your throat or on your tongue is the easiest way to feel good.

If you're looking for a beauty fix
There are a ton of deeply moisturizing and inflammation-fighting CBD face creams, eye rollers, soaps, and other beauty products on the market. Kana Skincare's CBD Korean sleeping mask is light enough to use every night and is

formulated by a grandma in Seoul who makes high-end beauty creams.

If you're craving a delicious treat
CBD chocolate, gummies, granola bars, and even cotton candy are the perfect snack that you can justify as (somewhat) "healthy" for you.

If your pet wants a treat too
CBD pet tinctures are often infused with good stuff like cod liver oil and omega-3 fatty acids to keep your pooch's fur shiny—because they deserve to look as good as they feel. If you have an anxious feline friend, a drop of hemp oil made for cats should help to get it purring in no time.

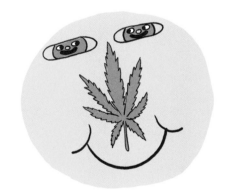

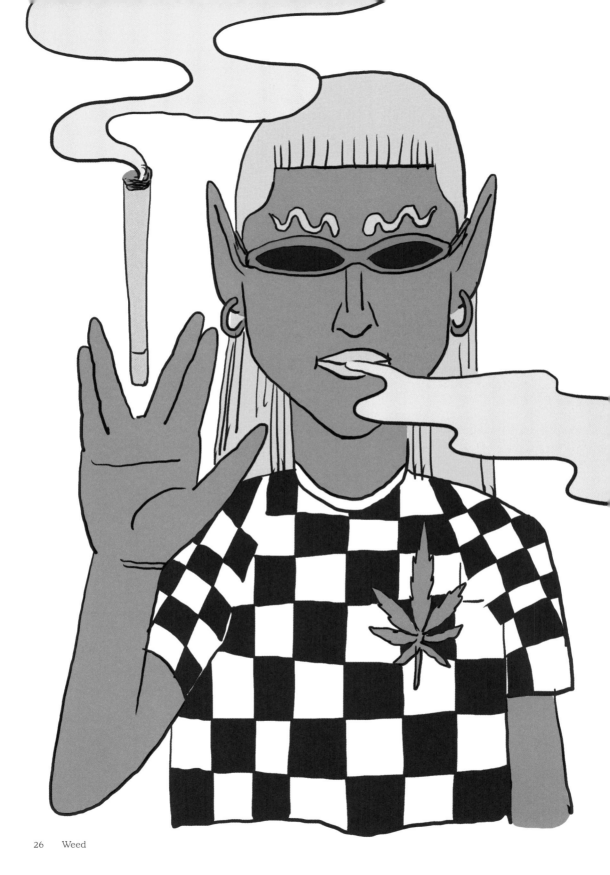

The Next Generation

While THC and CBD are currently hogging the limelight, a weed plant contains at least eighty-five known cannabinoids (some people say closer to a hundred), and a bunch of others are now on the up. Research into these cannabinoids is still pretty limited but there have been exciting signs in terms of their possible medical uses, including potentially helping to fight cancer, diabetes, and depression. You can't really buy these cannabinoids in flower form yet, but you might be able to find them in dab oil (see p. 56) or vape cartridge form if you look hard enough.

Delta-8-THC
Good for: Getting stoned but not *too* stoned

A close cousin to the THC everyone knows (which is technically delta-9-THC), delta-8 is found in very small amounts in the cannabis plant. You'll still get stoned, but the high will be a little more subtle and mellow, and it tastes a bit sweeter.

THCV
Good for: Curbing munchie cravings

One of the most annoying side effects of weed is waking up in a pile of junk-food wrappers. THCV is the anti-munchies savior—it actually kills your appetite, while giving you a boost of energy and a nice stoned buzz. THCV is most abundant in sativas, especially strains from Africa like Durban Poison. Many cannabis brands and pharmaceutical companies have already latched on to this cannabinoid; research suggests it could help fight panic attacks, prevent seizures, stimulate bone growth, and treat diet-related conditions like type 2 diabetes.

CBN
Good for: Beauty sleep

You know how you get sleepy after smoking stale weed? That's because of CBN, or cannabinol, which is what THCA breaks down into over time and exposure to oxygen. For a long time CBN was seen as "the enemy" because it's a sign that weed has gone bad. But it might help to soothe muscles, reduce pain, and fight signs of aging, making it a popular contender for use in weed beauty products.

THCA
Good for: "Wellness"

The cannabis plant actually doesn't contain THC—it contains THCA, or tetrahydrocannabinolic acid, an inactive compound that won't get you stoned. Through a process called "decarboxylation," usually achieved through heating up weed with a lighter, vape, or oven (see p. 68), THCA gets converted into THC. Thus THCA is a good way to absorb the physical benefits of pot without any psychoactive effects, sort of similar to CBD. It can help to regulate your immune and hormone systems and might even help to prevent the spread of cancer. You can find THCA sold as patches or other topicals that you apply to your skin, as well as in capsules that you swallow. If you're growing your own cannabis plants at home, you can juice the leaves to drink up this good stuff.

CBG
Good for: Low mood; high blood pressure

CBG, or cannabigerol, is known as the "mother" of cannabinoids, since the plant produces a lot of it and then converts it into all the others. It may be useful as an antidepressant, muscle relaxant, antibiotic, and antifungal agent. It may also help reduce blood pressure.

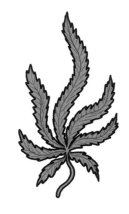

TERPENES

Have you ever wondered why Sour Diesel tastes different from Lemon Haze? Or why you prefer one strain over another, even if they have similar names or the same THC levels? Maybe you've never thought about it that much, or just assumed that's how the ganja gods meant for it to be. But the answer—at least partly—is terpenes.

Terpenes are the essential oils of the cannabis plant. There are over a hundred known cannabis terpenes, and each strain has a unique combination of them, giving it a distinctive smell and flavor. But it's not just about aromatics. Like cannabinoids, terpenes are stored in the trichome glands of the cannabis plant, and they help to mediate how our bodies interact with weed. Some terpenes relieve stress, while others increase focus or elevate mood. Certain terpenes might even reduce the harm caused to your lungs by inhaling cannabis smoke—a fact that low-key blew my mind when I first found out about it.

Recently, as the average stoner has become more aware of what terpenes do, public interest has spiked. The word "terpene" is now Googled about five times more regularly than it was two or three years ago. Weed strains and concentrates high in naturally derived terpenes are now extremely popular. When you see a cannabis product advertised as "full spectrum," that usually means that the grower or extractor made an effort to maximize its terpenes and cannabinoids in order to create a well-rounded high that feels as good as it tastes.

Thus, knowing which terpenes you like (or want to avoid) will really help you in choosing the right strains for you. Though, if you're ever in doubt, just take a deep whiff and trust your nose, because chances are that your subconscious instincts will guide you to what your body needs the most.

Popular Terpenes

Myrcene
Aroma: Musky and earthy, with a hint of floral
Effects: That relaxed feeling of not wanting to get off your butt, also known as "couch lock"
Strains: Pure Kush; White Widow

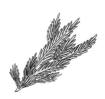

Pinene
Aroma: Pine and fir
Effects: Keeping you alert; fighting germs; helping your lungs stay clear
Strains: Jack Herer; Durban Poison

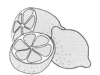

Limonene
Aroma: Lemon and orange
Effects: Uplifting your mood; giving you a burst of energy; curbing your appetite
Strains: Super Lemon Haze; Lemon Skunk

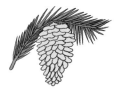

Terpineol
Aroma: Pine and clove
Effects: Antioxidant
Strains: OG Kush; Girl Scout Cookies

Borneol
Aroma: Menthol
Effects: Chilling you out and helping you de-stress
Strains: K13; Sour Diesel

Delta-3-Carene
Aroma: Sweet and musky
Effects: Cottonmouth and red eyes
Strains: Super Silver Haze; Skunk #1

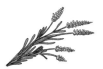

Linalool
Aroma: Floral and lavender
Effects: Soothes anxiety
Strains: G-13; Amnesia Haze

INTERVIEW WITH WEED SOMMELIER JAMIE EVANS

Imagine you're at a fancy restaurant. A waiter approaches your table. "May I recommend our Northern Lights strain?" she says, holding up a vape pen for your inspection. "It's our 2016 vintage, with clove and black pepper aromas, and will pair *excellently* with your steak." It might sound wild, but weed sommeliers are already carving out a niche in the industry. And according to Jamie Evans, founder of online guide *The Herb Somm*, public demand for their expertise is going to keep growing as legal cannabis spreads around the world.

Evans is a self-trained weed sommelier with a long background in the world of wine. She started her company in 2017, sharing cannabis recipes on her website and throwing gourmet weed-and-wine dinners with names like "Terpenes and Terroir" in the Bay Area. In between jetting around the US for extravagant dinner parties, she gave me the scoop on the life of a weed sommelier.

What does it take to be a weed sommelier?
A great nose and palate, and a lot of attention to detail. I spent over ten years in the wine industry

developing my senses of smell and taste. I use similar sensory evaluation techniques for cannabis and wine—it's all about using your natural senses to determine quality. It's also important to be able to pick out flaws in your cannabis, and to be able to make recommendations based on someone's needs. If you aspire to be a weed connoisseur, you better know your shit!

Why should we care about terpenes, and how exactly do they work?
Terpenes help us better understand cannabis's impact on the human body. We can use cannabis more effectively by learning what each terpene can do. Cannabis plants are packed with different aromas, flavors, and therapeutic properties. Each strain has different cannabinoid and terpene profiles due to farming practices and the terroir in which it was grown.

Produced in the same gland as the cannabinoids THC and CBD, terpenes are chemical compounds that give cannabis their aromas and flavors. They have many health benefits, including reducing inflammation, stress, and anxiety. Terpenes also

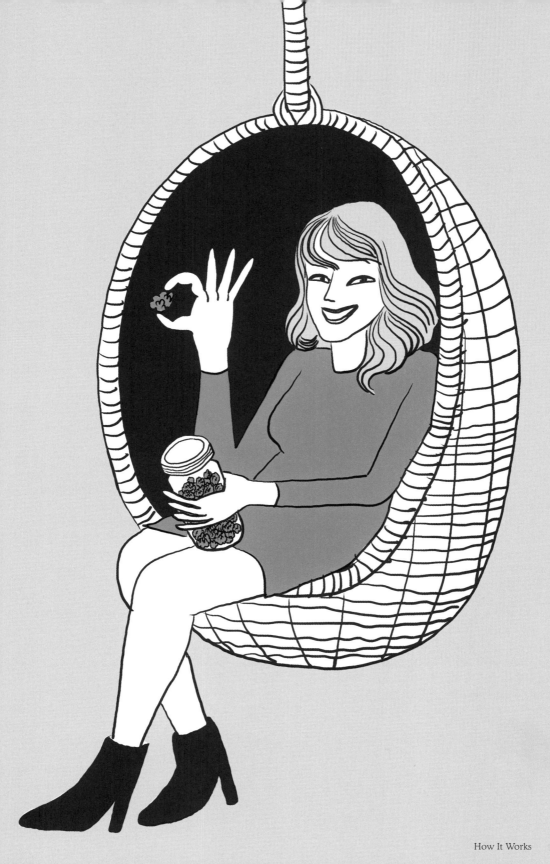

interact synergistically with cannabinoids to create what researchers call the "ensemble" or "entourage effect" (see p. 18). Due to these interactions, certain strains will make you feel uplifted, sleepy, energized, and so on.

Can the smell of weed give you an indication of what consuming it will feel like?

Absolutely! This is the beauty of understanding terpene profiles. For example, if you're smelling a strain that has notes of lemon, lime, grapefruit, or tangerine, you will most likely feel uplifted, refreshed, and energized. This is due to the citrusy terpene limonene. This terpene also reduces stress, promotes weight loss, and fights depression.

Do weed sommeliers describe weed the way wine folks do, like, "It has a hint of grass, with notes of pine"?

I don't know about other people, but I certainly do! Here's a tasting note I wrote on Humboldt Farms' Blue Dream strain:

"Blue Dream is a cross of Blueberry indica and Haze sativa. This hybrid strain has lovely notes of red raspberry, blueberry, floral spice, and earth (similar to Syrah and Grenache). A slight citrus characteristic is also perceived in the upper nostrils. This strain is very balanced and enhances full body relaxation. It's also one of California's most popular strains. Because it is a hybrid, it will pair well with rosé wines, which are also very versatile for any occasion. This strain is highest in linalool and caryophyllene terpenes, delivering fresh floral and spice notes."

Terpenes have become a really hot topic among stoners in recent years. What impact do you think this is having?

The discovery of terpenes is helping the cannabis industry rebrand itself. It's not just about sativa and indica anymore. Terpene research has also become more accessible in recent years, but we're still at the tip of the iceberg. Federal prohibition has slowed scientific research compared to countries ahead of the curve, including Israel and Spain. As we continue to learn more about the benefits of each terpene and how they affect the human body, we'll discover even more remarkable uses for cannabis.

Weed sommeliers have been in the news a lot lately. Why do you think this field is booming?

It's a great time to be a weed sommelier. Not many people specialize in this field, so there are opportunities to spread knowledge and make a name for yourself. Excellent weed sommelier programs are also now available, particularly the Trichome Institute's Interpening program. I've seen a lot of budtenders and chefs take this course [so that they can] make accurate recommendations or gourmet infusions. As laws continue to change, the weed sommelier will be just as respected and prevalent as the wine sommelier. People love learning from experts.

What should you expect from a terpene training course?

Basically, an interpening course will show you how to use your senses to assess a plant's terpenes and flower structure, inspect bud quality, and predict effects. Because of my extensive background in wine, I never took a formal weed sommelier course. Instead, I trained myself by going to dispensaries and learning about strains from budtenders, or examining, smelling, and tasting on my own. I did, however, purchase the Trichome Institute's Interpening guide book, which taught me the basics.

How can a weed sommelier use their skills to find work?

If you're planning to be a budtender, cannabis chef, or educator, you'll be using your weed sommelier skills a lot. If you have an entrepreneurial spirit, you could also find a niche market and launch your own business. My business has been successful because I specialize in cannabis and wine pairings, as well as pairing cannabis with different foods. Once cannabis becomes federally legal in the US, I think we'll see the rise of the cannabis restaurant. This will be a fantastic opportunity for weed sommeliers, giving them a platform to showcase what they can do.

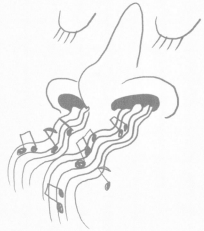

How to Train Your Nose, According to *The Herb Somm*

These techniques work for both cannabis and wine sommelier training!

1. "Take mental notes on the aromas around you. Pay attention to the foods that you eat, and the aromas and flavors that stand out. Also, learn about terpene profiles and the common aromas associated with each."

2. "The next time you're in the kitchen, go to your spice rack and pull out a selection to smell and taste. Start with herbs and spices that have similar terpene aromas as cannabis, like rosemary, black pepper, dill, oregano, cinnamon, nutmeg, and clove. Close your eyes, inhale deeply from each jar one at a time, and make a mental imprint of what you're smelling."

3. "Head to the grocery store and pick up foods commonly mentioned in cannabis descriptions, like lemons, grapefruits, blueberries, mushrooms, lavender, strawberries, fresh herbs, and mango. When you get home, cut up or muddle the items separately, place them into small jars or glasses, and smell the aromas. Don't forget to take a bite—especially if you have the munchies."

4. "Now apply what you've learned to cannabis. Put different strains of cannabis in individual jars, and keep the jars closed until you're ready to smell them. If you don't have access to different strains at home, head to your local dispensary and ask the budtender if you can smell a selection. Think about what you're smelling: are any of the aromas familiar? If so, you've successfully trained your nose to identify aromas."

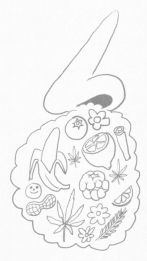

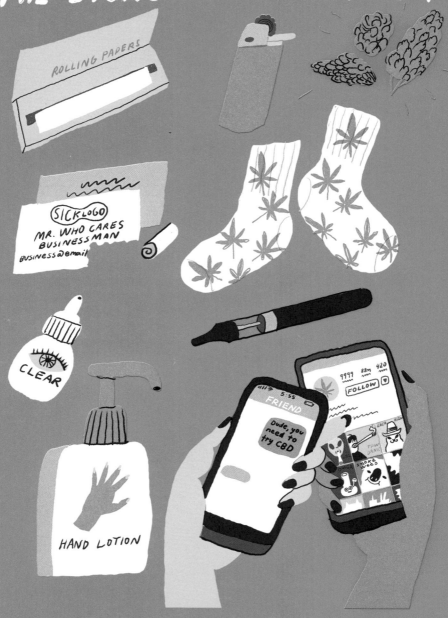

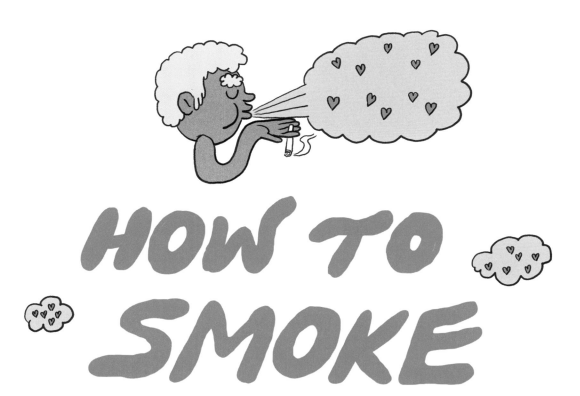

HOW TO SMOKE

Now for the fun part: how to get stoned. There are a dizzying number of ways to smoke weed, but I like to think this vast cosmos can be boiled down into two camps: old-school (joints, blunts, pipes, bongs), and new-school (vapes and dab rigs). Every method has its pros and cons—some are good for sharing with friends at parties, for example, while others are best left at home. What it comes down to is assessing what works best for whatever situation you find yourself in. Choose wisely, and you're the hero chilling by the pool bestowing everyone with a hit of your immaculately rolled joint. Miscalculate, and

you're the weirdo trying to sneak a butane torch into the club to dab on the dance floor.

Once you figure out what you like, it's easy to become a creature of habit and stick to the tried-and-true. But the world of cannabis is too diverse to limit yourself because you're afraid of trying something new. Maybe it's best to think of smoking weed like dating: why settle for something predictable when you can have more fun playing the field?

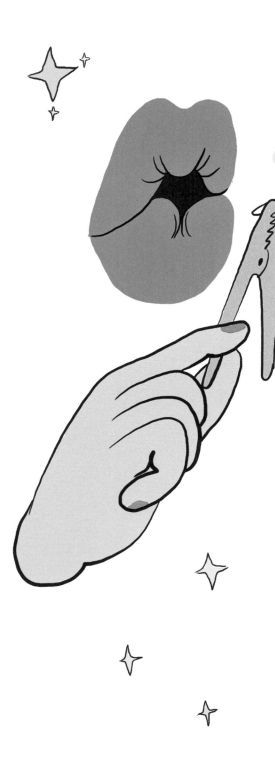

JOINTS

Show me your joint, and I'll tell you how you live. Like any art form, rolling a joint is an expression of who you are. Type As like to roll them straight and narrow; shy and quiet people tend to produce tiny little ones; while hedonists stuff them decadently into fatties.

Beautiful joints come in all shapes and sizes—there's no formula for perfection. The most important quality is that it smokes evenly without one side burning faster than the other. Everything else is aesthetic: how fat the joint is, the size of the filter, and the width of its conical shape are all up to you. A truly supreme joint, to nitpickers, is rolled with such skill that there are no wrinkles in the paper.

There are also many different ways that you can customize your joint. The most popular modification is called the "L," where you combine two papers at a ninety-degree angle to make an extra-long joint—best for when you're smoking with a big crew. One of my friends rolls his with super-long filters, making him look as elegant as Audrey Hepburn with her cigarette holder in *Breakfast at Tiffany's*. There's even a whole subculture of hardcore stoners who compete to make the craziest-shaped joints—smokable sculptures that look like octopuses, helicopters, or Christmas trees.

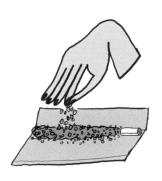
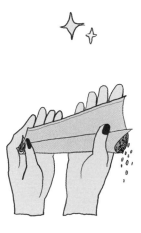
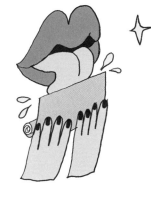

Hot Tips for Perfect Joints

1. Get primo papers
Go with organic or non-processed paper—
the thinner the better—so you're not inhaling
a bunch of crap.

2. Make a crutch
Some people don't use crutches (filters). These
people are usually hippies or wasteful hedonists
and should never be trusted. You can make
a good crutch by ripping off a thin piece of
cardboard (a ticket stub or cheap business card is
perfect), folding one end forward, then rolling it
backwards so that the ends make a Z-shape. This
gives it a nice form that air can flow through.

3. Add herbs
Herbs like lavender and sage can enhance the
taste and buzz of your joint, while also helping you
conserve weed.

4. Lick your fingers
If the paper feels kind of slippery, licking your
fingers a little will give you a better grip. Just
don't slobber all over them because it'll make
the paper break.

5. Pack the joint tight
Make sure the weed is packed tightly by twisting
the far end closed, then shaking it down from
the top.

6. Push the filter further into the joint
This is another great way to get rid of any
remaining air gaps.

7. Wet your canoe
If your joint starts to burn more quickly on one
side—a common pitfall called "canoeing"—lick
your finger and hold it briefly to the faster-burning
end. Act fast, or you could waste the whole joint.

8. Don't freak out
Rolling gets easier every time you do it, so don't
give up on learning this essential life skill. Maybe
watch some YouTube videos about it. You'll be
twisting joints standing up while chatting to cuties
on a roiling dance floor in no time.

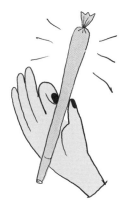

Types of Joints

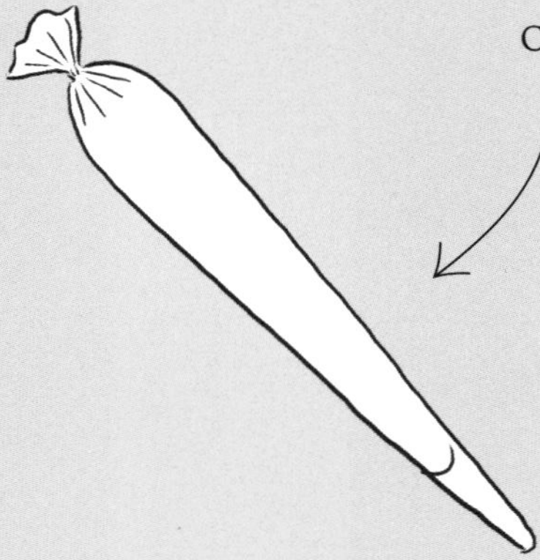

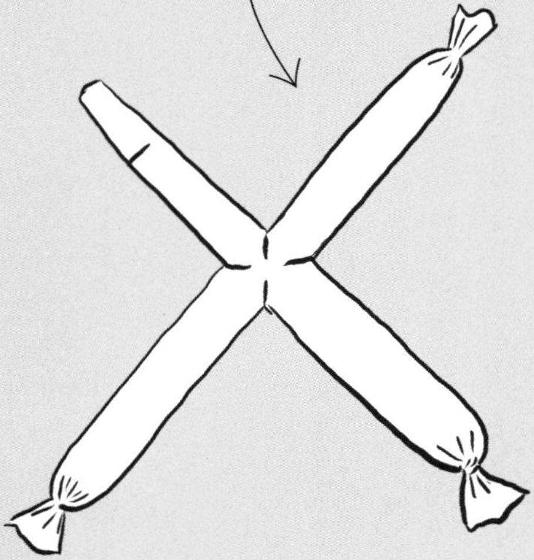

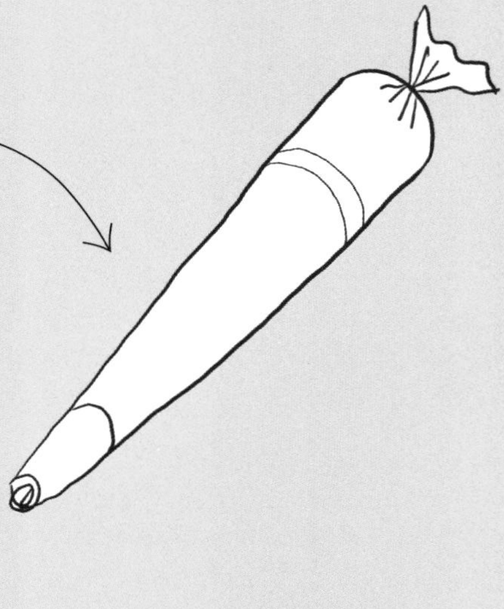

Cone

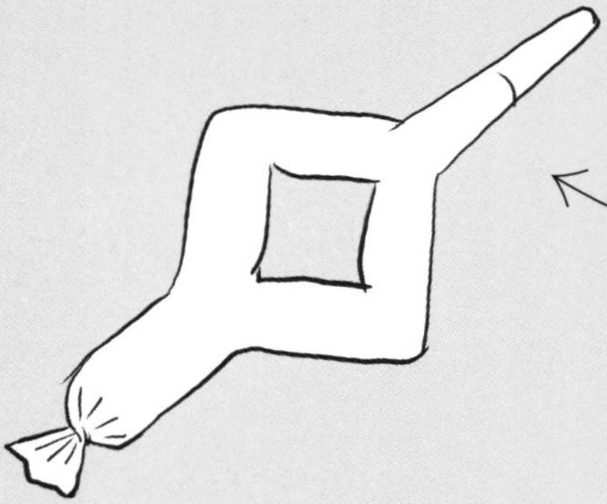

Diamond

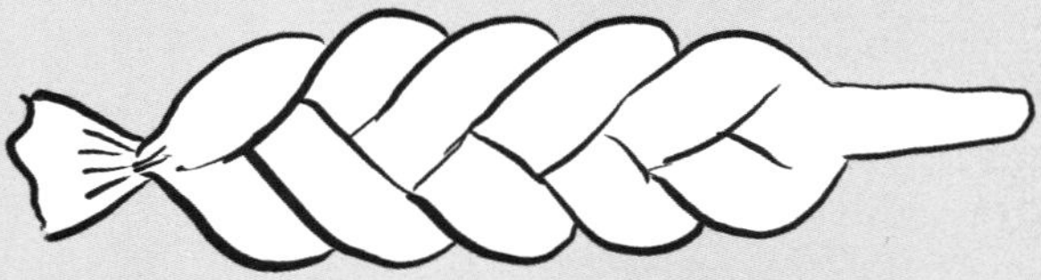

Cross

Braid

L

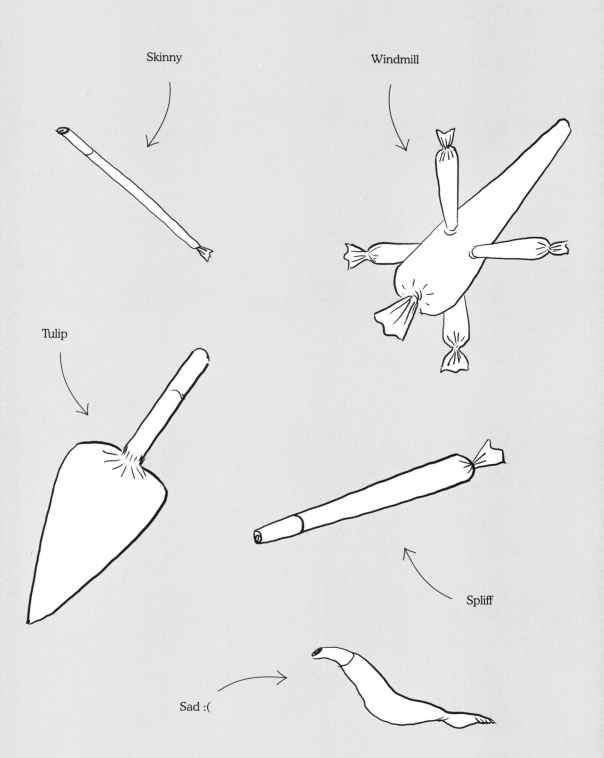

Skinny

Windmill

Tulip

Spliff

Sad :(

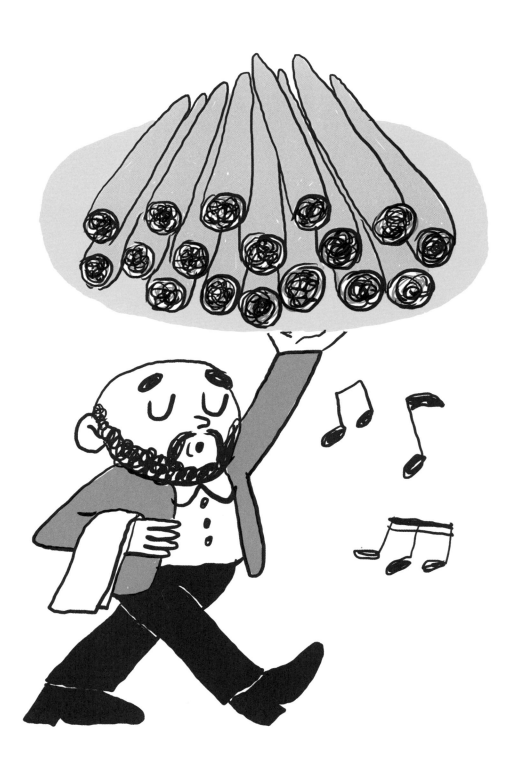

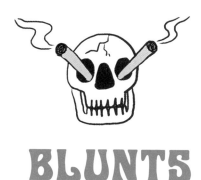

BLUNTS

Blunts are the most baller way to smoke weed. Filling a blunt wrap (the tobacco-leaf skin of a cigar) requires a ton of flower—so yeah, it's a bit wasteful—but showing off how much green you have to burn is precisely the point, and part of the reason why fat blunts are status symbols. If a joint is like a cannabis cigarette, then a blunt is a weed cigar. They're thicker, more expensively indulgent, and likely to be richer in taste thanks to the variety of flavors you can get blunt wraps in (strawberry is a classic). Plus, the tobacco from the leaf will make you feel extra-buzzy and ready to party.

While pipes and bongs are sometimes associated with hippie culture from the 1970s, blunts were popularized in the early '80s. "I love it when they call me Big Poppa / I only smoke blunts if they rolled proper," rapped Biggie in the '90s. You could say that blunts are hip-hop's favorite muse: Nas got existential about the ephemerality of life on "Blunt Ashes," Missy Elliot wanted you to "Pass That Dutch," 50 Cent was "High All the Time," Danny Brown was going "Blunt After Blunt" … hell, Snoop Dogg's entire career is based on getting stoned.

Historically, blunt preferences in America were tied to where you were from. The West Coast swore allegiance to the Swisher Sweets brand, while East Coasters preferred Dutch Masters and White Owl. The Phillies brand was tied to Philadelphia, naturally, while Southern cities like Atlanta became associated with Backwoods.

These days, with everyone flexing their blunt game on social media, geography-based allegiances have been, at least among hardcore blunt heads, replaced by the allure of rare super-blunts. Cool, cred-seeking smokers will even pay up to $45 for rare and vintage grape, banana, or vanilla-flavored Backwoods on eBay, packing their blunts with an eighth of weed (for some people, an entire week's stash) so they can stunt on Instagram.

Still, blunts are just as—if not more—popular today as they were back when Biggie was rapping about how much smoke was coming out of his nose. Culture changes, but one thing will always remain the same: there's no better way to signal that you're a baller than smoking a fattie blunt.

How to Roll a Blunt Like a Boss

Rolling a blunt isn't terribly different from rolling a joint—it just requires a few more steps, an extra bit of effort … and a lot more weed. Luckily, Def Jam rapper Redman dropped all the info you need to follow in an iconic 1992 track called "How to Roll a Blunt." Since there's no one better to explain this glorified ritual, here's an annotated version of his lyrics:

1. **"First of all, you get a fat bag of ism"**
Get yourself a ton of weed.

2. **"From Uptown, any local store sells the shit, friend / Purchase a Phillie—not the city of Philly, silly punk / I'm talking about the cigar, the Phillie Blunt"**
Blunts originally got their name from the Phillies Blunt cigar, although these days there are tons of different cigar types to choose from, including hollow blunt wraps that save you the trouble of having to empty out tobacco. Hit up your local smoke shop and look for popular brands like Swisher Sweets, Phillies, or Backwoods.

3. **"Lick the blunt …"**
Wet the leaf by licking it all over, or by dipping your fingers in water if you're sharing with someone who cares about "germs." You can also wrap it in a moist paper towel for a few seconds. Making sure the cigar is moist is really important for ensuring it doesn't crack at any point and sticks together properly.

4. **"… and then the Phillie Blunt middle you split / Don't have a razor blade, use your fuckin' fingertips"**
Split the cigar using a sharp edge like a blade or your fingernails, cracking it open vertically starting from the side where your mouth will go and working your way up to the end that will be lit. Empty out the tobacco.

5. **"Crack the bag and then you pour the whole bag in / Spread the ism around until the ism reach each end"**
Fill the wrap with a gram or two of ground-up weed (more if you're feeling decadent).

6. **"Take your finger and your thumb from tip to tip / Roll it in a motion, then the top piece you lick"**
Roll up the blunt following the same steps as with a joint, working your way to the final fold.

7. **"Seal it, dry it wit ya lighter if ya gotta"**
Seal it up by licking the inside of the exposed side from end to end before you tuck it. Bake the blunt by waving a lighter flame along it from end to end, which helps dry it out and seal it up. Careful not to hold the lighter too close or the blunt will get scorched.

8. **"The results, mmmmmmmm … proper"**
Light up and lean back.

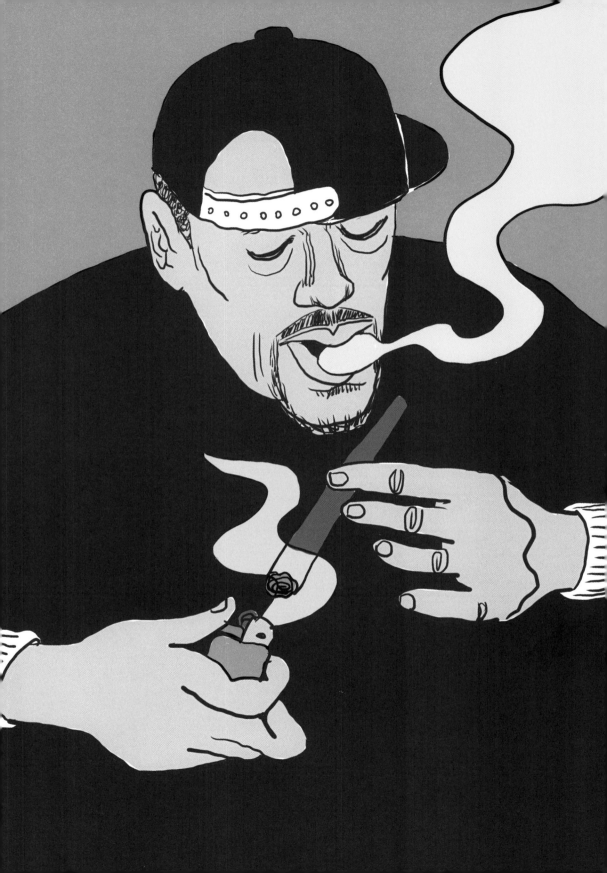

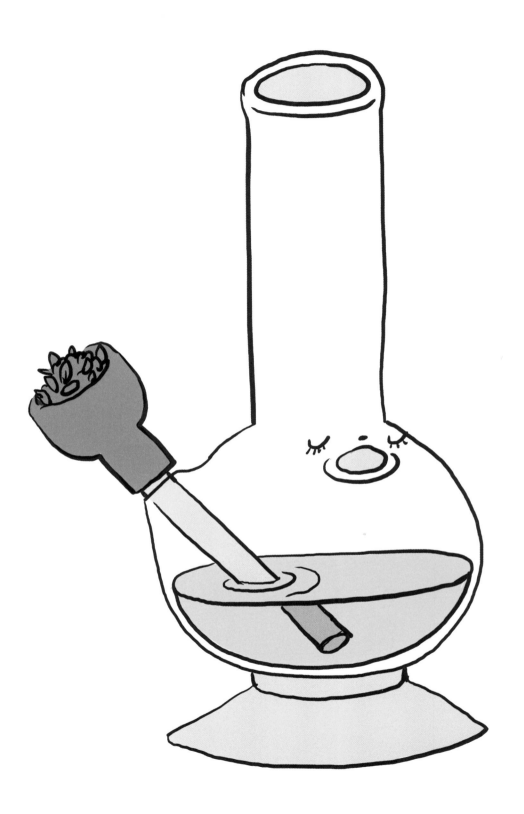

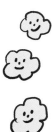

BONGS

Wanna smoke a bowl? Then get yourself a pipe or bong, classic cannabis contraptions that every stoner should have on their shelf. Bongs date all the way back to 2,400 years ago, when they were used by chiefs of the Scythian tribe in what's now Russia. Specimens from around 1100 CE made out of animal horns and pottery have been found in an ancient Ethiopian cave, while bamboo was the material of choice for bongs in sixteenth-century Central Asia; in fact, the word "bong" comes from the Thai word buang, meaning bamboo pipe. The ingenious idea of filling bongs with water was invented by the Chinese during the Ming dynasty (1368–1644), spreading throughout the continent via the Silk Road. The Empress Dowager Cixi, who controlled the Qing dynasty for five decades, was even buried with three of her favorite bongs when she died in 1908.

These days, bongs have evolved to suit every kind of stoner. If you're a tech nerd getting high to episodes of Silicon Valley, there are futuristic contraptions that look like the kinds of bongs that stoner aliens might pass around a crop circle, boasting an array of digital functions like precise heat control via a phone app. If you're a vegan in Brooklyn who likes your juice to be cold-pressed with a dash of activated charcoal, you can decorate your coffee table with a refined, modern bong that looks like a multitasking flower vase from the MoMA gift shop. These sleek bongs are like catnip to design-conscious hipsters repulsed by the "druggie" aesthetic of old-school hippie bongs.

Conversely, if you're actually into that psychedelic aesthetic, hand-blown artisanal glass bongs have also gone next-level, while recalling the thirteenth-century Venetian glass art tradition. Some collector's items are so gorgeous that art galleries have devoted entire exhibitions to them; an intricate, life-size skeleton-shaped masterpiece by legendary glass artist Kevin Murray went on sale for a cool million bucks at a Massachusetts art show in 2017.

Whatever type you choose, bongs are both statement pieces and a smooth way to get stoned. Since the smoke cools down as it travels through the piece, it's a little easier on your lungs than a joint or blunt. Plus, since you only burn what you inhale, you don't waste as much weed. Many potheads love their bongs so much they give them nicknames, so don't get weirded out if you hear someone referring to theirs like a loved one. After all, bongs really are a stoner's best friend.

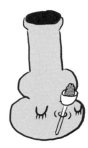

Anatomy of a Bong

Base
Comes in several different shapes, including straight-tube, beaker, and round. A beaker base that's flared at the end is less likely to tip over and can contain more water than a straight-tube base.

Water Chamber
The bottom area of the bong, which you fill with water.

Ice Pinch
Inward-facing points that let you fill the tube with ice to further cool down the smoke.

Tube
After the smoke passes through the water chamber, it flows up into the vertical tube towards the mouthpiece. Tubes can contain a variety of percolators to filter out the smoke.

Percolators ("Percs")
Chambers that help to filter and cool down the smoke. More complicated (read: expensive) bongs have fancy, multi-chamber percs to diffuse the smoke even further.

Bowl
The area where you pack in your weed.

Downstem
A long tube connected to the bowl that allows smoke to flow through the water chamber, producing a lighter and smoother hit.

Carb
A small hole above the water line that you cover with your thumb as you inhale, then release so that fresh air flows in. Not all bongs have carbs.

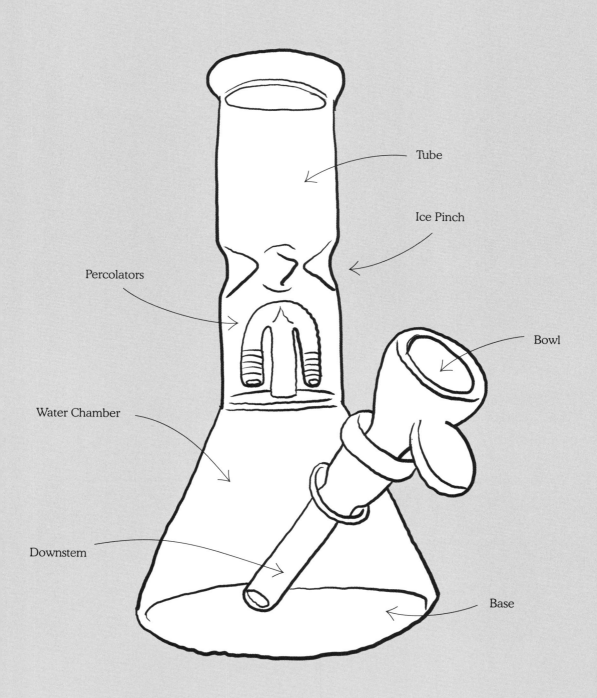

Tube

Ice Pinch

Percolators

Bowl

Water Chamber

Downstem

Base

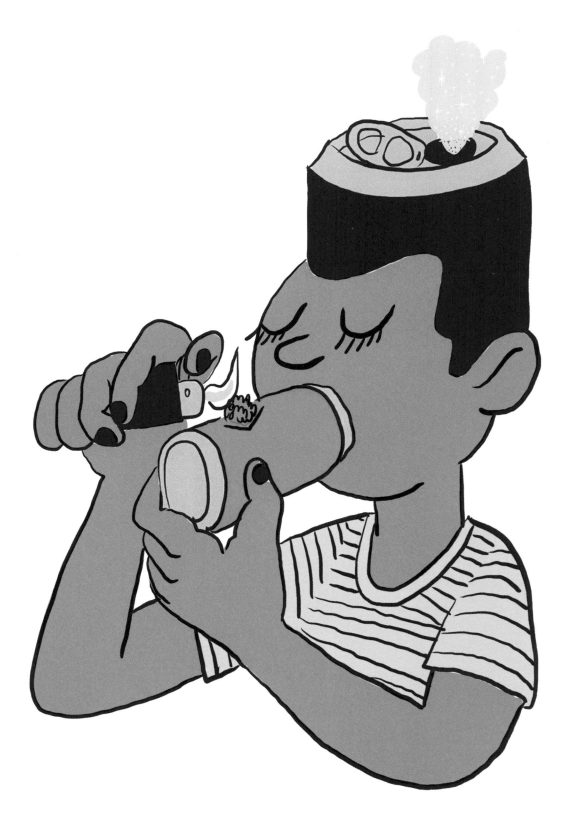

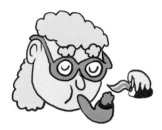

PIPES

Just like bongs, pipes have helped people get baked for centuries. Lengthy wooden pipes known as "sebsis" have long been the traditional way to smoke hash in Morocco, while small, conical clay versions called "chillums" have been used by Hindu monks in India since at least the eighteenth century. Recently, scientists discovered that four-hundred-year-old pipes excavated from Shakespeare's garden in Stratford-upon-Avon contained cannabis residue—suggesting that some of the greatest works in English literature were written stoned.

The psychedelic glass pipes you'll often find in college dorm rooms can be traced back to an artist named Bob Snodgrass. While following the Grateful Dead on tour in the 1970s and '80s, he invented a technique that allowed his pipes to change color, as resin built up along their insides the more you used them. Hippies and potheads of all kinds flocked to these vividly hued pieces, which became wildly popular and earned Snodgrass the nickname "godfather of modern glassblowing."

Soon, Tommy Chong—one half of the comedy duo Cheech & Chong—got in on the glass game, selling artisanal pipes and bongs decorated with a painted cartoon of his face, complete with his iconic round glasses and bandana. But in 2003 the Feds launched Operation Pipe Dreams, a $12 million crackdown on head shops selling drug paraphernalia. Among the people they arrested was Chong, who was sentenced to nine months in federal prison. As stoners across the world rallied around him, the crackdown's attempt to quash weed culture's beloved smoking accessories turned out to be, well, a pipe dream.

But while technicolored glass pieces still line the shelves of smoke shops everywhere, modern pipes are appealing to a new demographic of sophisticated smokers. Made in muted tones and using earthy materials like porcelain, New Agey crystals such as quartz, and stone, lots of today's pipes aren't something you need to stash out of sight in a drawer. Some even claim they're so beautiful that you wouldn't even dare to smoke out of them … Yeah, right.

Popular Pipes

Spoon Pipe

The most common type of pipe, marked by a bowl at the end of a neck that connects to the mouthpiece, and a "carb," an air hole that you have to plug up with your finger in order to draw the smoke into your lungs to take a hit.

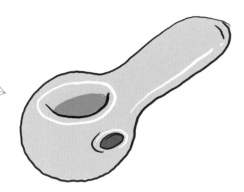

One-Hitter

A super-portable pipe that can only pack a little bit of weed; good for one or two hits. Often comes in small sizes and disguised to look like a cigarette just in case any narcs are lurking around.

Chillum

A simple tube-shaped pipe that dates back to eighteenth-century Hindu monks in India, who used them for spiritual and meditative practices. Usually has a bowl slightly larger than on a one-hitter.

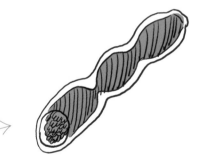

Monkey Pipe

Wooden pipes that can be swiveled closed from a hinge in the middle. They don't have a carb.

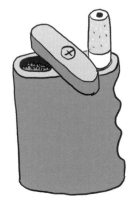

Chamber Pipe
Made from metal, these pipes have an air chamber connected to the bowl that helps to cool off the smoke before it reaches the mouthpiece.

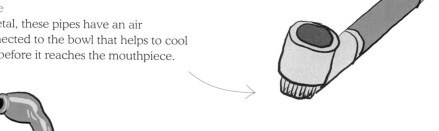

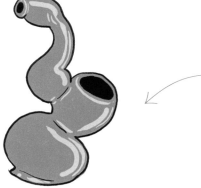

Bubbler
A cross between a regular pipe and a water bong, a bubbler lets you fill the bottom chamber with water for a way smoother hit.

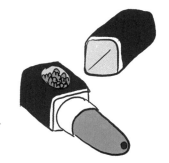

Stealth Pipe
A pipe sneakily disguised to look like a lipstick, a pen, a flashlight … anything but something you'd smoke weed with.

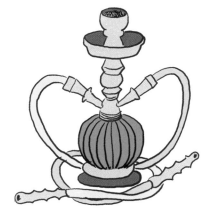

Hookah
A traditional water pipe for smoking hookah (flavored tobacco) that can also come in mini sizes and is an extravagant way to smoke either hash or weed.

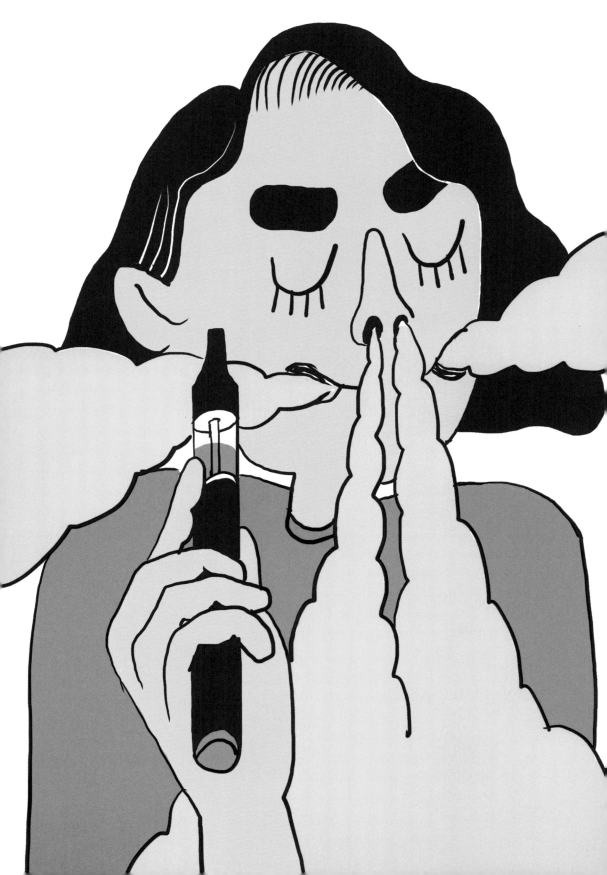

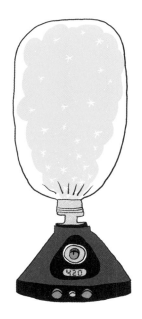

VAPES

Weed jumped from analog to digital when we went from joints to vapes. The transition was kind of like going from vinyl to mp3: maybe something raw was lost in our pursuit of convenience, but technology also opened up a brave new world of possibility. When those scentless clouds of vapor hit, it felt like a revelation. You could get stoned *anywhere* and not have to be that person awkwardly rolling a joint under the table, or anxiously puffing a one-hitter in the bathroom.

Vape technology has been around for longer than you might expect—the first electronic cigarette patent was filed in 1963. E-cigarettes really started catching on in the early 2000s, and digitizing weed was the next logical step. Early vapes started out kind of clunky—remember the Volcano, pictured above?—and were often too expensive to be really worth it. Many resembled a plastic brick and were easily mistaken for a walkie-talkie radio or Taser.

In the 2010s, smaller and more portable vapes like G Pens and the PAX became popular. Then weed pens started popping up everywhere. Finally, vapes that didn't weigh a ton or look like a steampunk vibrator!

The vape market has since exploded. Everyone is now hitting weed pens that charge via USB and let you screw in disposable, pre-filled cartridges of cannabis extract (single-use disposables are also super-trendy). Some vapes Bluetooth sync to your phone; others give you a light show on their LED displays. And while not too long ago vapes were seen as either a nerdy fetish or dumb trend, they're now the easiest way to get into pot if you're entry-level. It's official: #VAPELIFE is the new slogan of stoner culture.

Anatomy of a Vape Pen

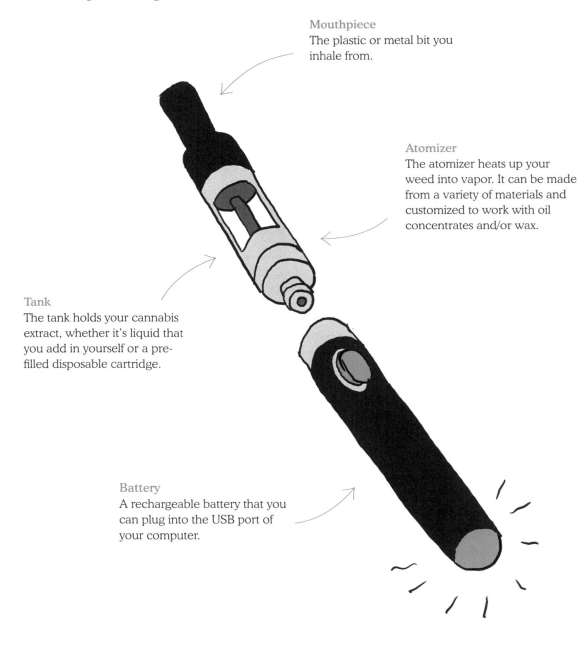

Mouthpiece
The plastic or metal bit you inhale from.

Atomizer
The atomizer heats up your weed into vapor. It can be made from a variety of materials and customized to work with oil concentrates and/or wax.

Tank
The tank holds your cannabis extract, whether it's liquid that you add in yourself or a pre-filled disposable cartridge.

Battery
A rechargeable battery that you can plug into the USB port of your computer.

How to Vape

Due to the dizzying levels of customizability and technology, discussions around vaping can turn into *heated* debates. We'll avoid this by simply recommending that you go down the easiest route: a vape pen.

First, choose a weed pen

Have you noticed how you sometimes sneeze after hitting a vape? That can be from too-hot oil scorching your pipes as you inhale. Studies also suggest that the hotter your vape gets, the more carcinogens you inhale. So the safest bet is to get a lower-voltage vape pen with several temperature controls.

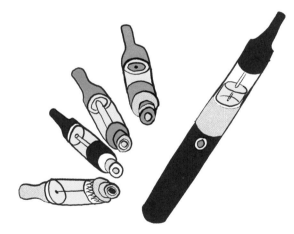

There are basically two types of vape pen: cartridge–battery combos that are sold separately, and disposables. Most batteries can be charged via USB and come in a standard format that works with any weed oil cartridge that you screw in. However, some vapes only work with the company's own customized cartridges. Disposables don't need to be charged at all—you just throw them out when they're out of juice. (This also makes them a great dinner party gift in lieu of wine.)

Then, get oiled up

Cannabis oils might look similar, but they're definitely not created equal. Lower-quality oils use scary extraction methods involving dangerous toxins like lighter fluid and additives—so you want to avoid these at all costs. Look for oils that say "CO_2" or "full-spectrum." Both of these indicate better extraction processes that allow oils to retain their terpenes—and this means they'll taste better, too.

An increasingly popular trend is for weed oils to be labeled by their intended mood, like "relaxing" or "uplifted," instead of a particular strain name. These oils are formulated using specific terpene combinations that are meant to produce certain effects. While the accuracy of these stated effects is debatable, more terpenes is always better than none.

Honestly, both cannabis oils and vape technology are still in their early stages, and until there's better government regulation of how they're made and advertised, it's all a bit of a crapshoot—so read labels to be aware of what you're vaping, and stay away from the cheap stuff.

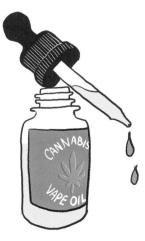

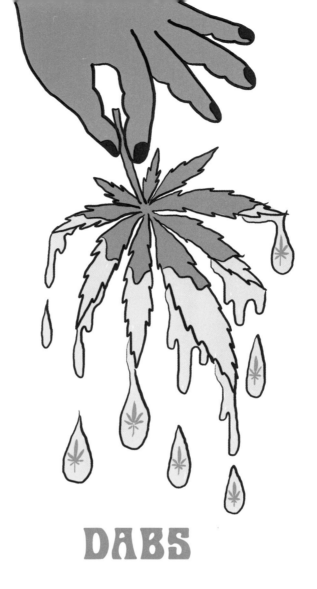

DABS

Concentrates, also known as "dabs" or "710," are cannabis extracts with potent levels of THC and other cannabinoids and terpenes. If puffing on a weed pen is like sipping a beer, then dabbing is like slamming a triple shot of vodka. You'll need a "dab rig"—essentially, a type of bong made for concentrates. Since waxes and oils need to be heated to extremely high temperatures in order to turn into vapor, a simple lighter isn't going to cut it: you're going to need a butane torch. If wielding a giant blowtorch sounds terrifying, get your hands on a more advanced, electronic dab rig instead.

Dabbing used to be an underground activity among hardcore stoners, who would make their own dab rigs by modifying traditional bongs. But in the mid-2000s, as people became increasingly concerned over inhaling smoke toxins, dabbing started to enter the mainstream, with a variety of increasingly sophisticated rigs flooding the market.

While it might seem a little intimidating at first, dabbing is the cleanest and most effective way to get extremely stoned very quickly. There are lots of different consistencies of concentrates, and they can contain as much as 70 to 90 percent THC, so start with a small dose as you work your way up to weed heaven.

Anatomy of a Dab Rig

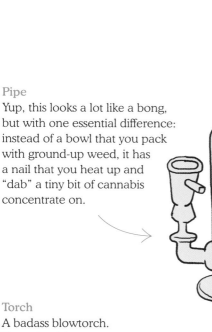

Pipe

Yup, this looks a lot like a bong, but with one essential difference: instead of a bowl that you pack with ground-up weed, it has a nail that you heat up and "dab" a tiny bit of cannabis concentrate on.

Dome

An (optional) additional piece that goes over the nail in order to trap the vapor while you're inhaling.

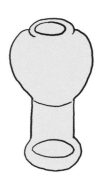

Torch

A badass blowtorch. Enough said.

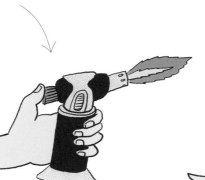

Nail

Without a doubt the most important part of a dab rig is the quality of the nail. Nails can be made from a variety of different materials, but the best ones are usually quartz or titanium as they're less likely to break than glass, which is also commonly used. There are also electronic nails for torch-free dabbing.

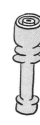

Wand

A utensil for picking up concentrates; comes in a variety of shapes.

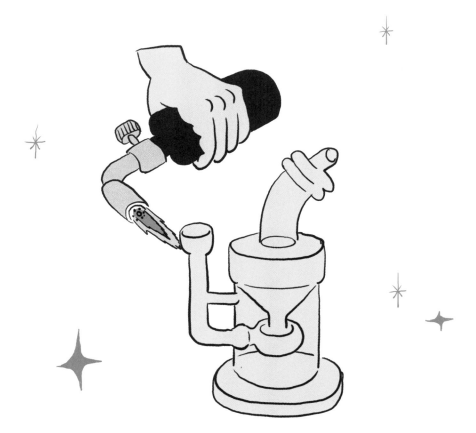

How to Dab

1. Heat the nail evenly with your torch (or electronically if using an e-nail). It's worth taking the time to read the manufacturer's specifications on how to handle the torch safely. Always make sure the flame points away from your pipe, or it might crack the glass.

2. Remove the flame once the nail starts to glow orange. If you have a dome, place it over the nail to maintain the temperature for as long as possible without having to add more heat.

3. As a good rule of thumb, wait 15 to 30 seconds for the nail to cool down slightly. If it's still glowing red, that's definitely too hot. Optimal temperatures for dabbing are *hotly* debated, but most experts recommend 500 to 540 degrees Fahrenheit (260 to 282 degrees Celsius). Keep in mind that the ideal temperature also varies based on what type of concentrate and nail you're using—and how stoned you want to get.

4. Use your dab tool or wand to scoop up a bit of concentrate, or if it's dry and crumbly enough, just break off a small piece with your fingers. Start with something about half the size of a grain of rice if you're a beginner.

5. Place the concentrate on the heated nail, rubbing your wand around the interior edges to spread it out evenly. It should release white wisps of vapor immediately.

6. Take a hit the same way you would from a bong, inhaling slowly but sharply enough to make the water bubble. Don't try to hold a dab hit in your lungs unless they're made of steel.

7. Inhale and exhale until you've had enough, or there's no more vapor left in the pipe's chamber. Chill for at least 15 minutes before taking another dab.

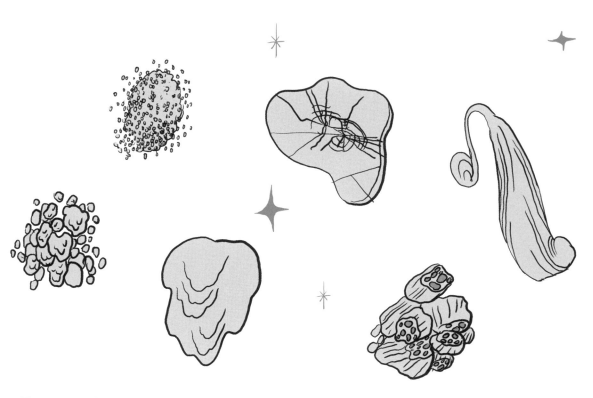

Types of Concentrates

Concentrates take on lots of different names depending on their consistency and extraction method. It can get pretty crazy out there, but here are several of the most common types of concentrates you'll encounter as you enter the wild world of dabbing:

Shatter
Looks like a sheet of transparent glass and has a reputation for being among the cleanest types of extract.

Wax
This one gets its name because it sort of looks like ear wax. There are many subtypes of wax depending on consistency, such as the creamy, butter-like "budder" and the more dry and brittle "honeycomb" or "crumble."

Rosin
While most extracts are made using some kind of chemical solvent, rosin is produced through a combination of heat and pressure—usually by smashing a nug of weed with a hair straightener. This produces an oil-like extract with nice, potent flavors.

Sap
A runny substance that looks like maple syrup.

Pull-and-Snap
Malleable oils that fall between shatter and sap.

Crystalline
The purest type of cannabis concentrate, crystalline looks like a shimmering crystal rock and usually consists of a single type of cannabinoid. THC-A crystallines are especially popular among dab heads thanks to its 99.9 percent THC content.

Oils
Typically made using CO_2 or butane, cannabis oils are most often found in vape pens and have runny, oily textures.

HOW TO MAKE ROSIN WITH FLOUR CHILD

Rosin is a type of weed concentrate made by applying so much intense pressure and heat to a cannabis flower that it secretes its oil, which you can then use for dabs. In the past few years, rosin has soared in popularity because, unlike extraction processes using butane or propane, this method preserves the plant's natural terpenes and cannabinoids without adding any icky chemicals. While professionals use expensive press machines, making rosin yourself is easy and quick—all you need is a piece of parchment paper to hold the bud, and a hair straightener to squish it with. (Although who owns a hair straightener these days? It's not the early 2000s.)

Stephany Gocobachi is the co-founder of Flour Child, a San Francisco-based company that sells granola and jams made with some of the best-tasting rosin in the game. A firm believer in organic and sustainable practices, Gocobachi is bringing the kind of farm-to-table attitude you'd find at a trendy rustic restaurant in Portland to the edibles industry. We spoke about how legalization is affecting small cannabis kitchens, the new school of edibles, and how to make the dankest rosin you've ever dabbed.

How did you get into making edibles?
I've been obsessed with food since I was a little kid in San Francisco, where cannabis was all around us. I started making edibles when I was sixteen, and when I went into a dispensary on my eighteenth birthday, I was so disappointed with what I saw on the shelves. Ten or twelve years ago, dosage wasn't even a consideration; the trend was to make everything as strong as possible. Nobody cared about ingredients or labeling. I had bought edibles on multiple occasions and gotten product that was moldy, stale, not labeled, and that, like, had pet hair in it—really egregious stuff.

It didn't make sense to me. If this was being sold as medicine, I didn't understand why it was all junk food made with shitty trim [low-quality weed] or really bad hash. All that did was perpetuate this negative stigma around cannabis. I didn't feel like it did anything to provide a service, or provide something of quality that would change the life of somebody who might benefit from it.

I went to New York University for college and started formulating a business plan, talking about it with my professors and classmates. At first I was very nervous to bring it up. I felt like it was sort of taboo—"is this okay to talk about?" But surprisingly it went over really well and sparked a lot of interest and curiosity. So I studied food sustainability and social entrepreneurship, because I felt like that would prepare me to run a really great edibles company. Then after I graduated I moved back to California and launched Flour Child.

Now, so many years later, cannabis is being treated like food and is regulated, so that's exciting and challenging at the same time for the industry. I think it's moving in the right direction. It's like if restaurants had never had to deal with a health department, and then all of a sudden there's a new health department that everyone has to deal with. I'm like, yay, finally we can be like a regular business—we can get real permits and be more open and transparent about it.

Your company is really into sustainable practices. How does that translate into edibles?
Farm-to-table and eating locally has become a very mainstream thing over the last few years, and I approach the cannabis that goes into my products like I approach any other ingredient. We try to source sun-grown, organic cannabis.

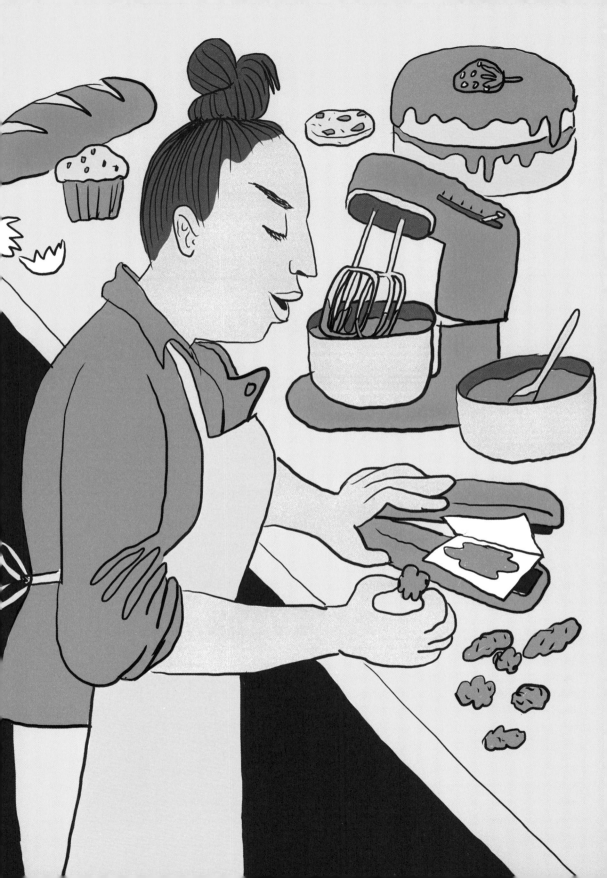

We always test everything before and after we process it. I like to develop relationships directly with farmers because I really believe in supporting people who are trying to run small businesses. I know what it's like, and how much of an impact it has if we support each other, versus buying factory-farm weed or food. It's all the same thing in my mind. It's better for you to source something that's been grown the way it was intended to be, not something that's artificially jacked up—even if it has a really high THC percentage, everything else is sucked out of it. It's like having a tomato in the summertime versus one that was grown in a hothouse 6,000 miles away. It tastes so different.

How does this organic philosophy connect to your use of rosin?
We press flowers using a little bit of heat and a lot of pressure to make our rosin. You can also press it out of hash extracted with cold water. Rosin is a more concentrated product that's solvent-free—I would never feed somebody butane or propane.

But it's really difficult to control the quality if you're not the one making it. So the goal was always to produce our own extracts, and we started pressing our own rosin so we could control what strains were going into it and what farms it was sourced from. And then we could offer rosin as its own [stand-alone] product.

The first couple times I got to cook with rosin, it was a dream to work with. With rosin, you just get the pure oil. It has a very beautiful fragrance; you get a clear expression of the plant without that really green, chlorophyll-y taste that people normally associate with edibles.

Something that a lot of people say when they try our products is, "Wow, it doesn't really taste like cannabis at all!" I'm like, "Well, you *can* taste it; it just tastes like good cannabis, not old moldy trim."

I like to make sure that our edibles are all very specific, because strains have different effects on different people. It's starting to change a little bit now, but there are still very few edibles out there that state what type of cannabis extract and strain they're made with.

How long has rosin been trendy for?
It's a very recent thing. Bubble hash [another type of cannabis concentrate] has been around for a long time. But the majority of what was out there before was all solvent-based extracts, like butane hash oil or propane hash oil, or with other hydrocarbon solvents. Rosin isn't an easy thing to find in shops, and I've gotten a few messages from people saying, like, "I usually only get BHO [butane hash oil] and it's hard to find rosin that's terpene-rich or as flavorful, but yours was the first one I've tried that I've actually liked." That always makes me do a little happy dance: when we can get a hardcore BHO person to enjoy rosin.

Rosin actually originated in the violin industry—they would catch animal fat or distill the resin from pine trees and use that to grease instruments. So if you say "rosin" to a musician, they're like, "for a string instrument?"

A couple of years ago, rosin got really popular via Instagram and YouTube. People started making rosin by taking a bud, putting it between parchment, and squishing it with a set of hair straighteners. It worked because making rosin is just a matter of pressing all the oils out and gathering it. In maybe the last two or three years, companies started to make actual presses for rosin as people started to figure out that they could do this commercially. It's picked up a lot in the dabbing community, because you can make a dab or concentrate at home without crazy equipment. And you can do it in really small batches, like one little bud at a time, and get a few dabs out of it.

Where do you think rosin is going next?
It's going to continue to grow a lot. Everybody is learning about it together. We're open about sharing information—like, we pressed *this* at *this* temperature for *this* many seconds, and *this* is what we got. In cannabis, there's a lot of secretiveness and everybody has a proprietary process. I'm all about empowering people. I don't have any secret recipes. I think it's better for everybody, for the industry and the consumers. I want everyone to make better products.

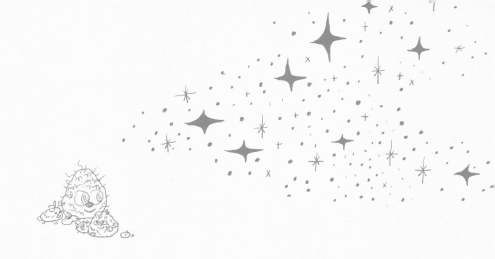

Rosin Tips from Flour Child

What you put in is what you'll get out
"It starts with the material that you use. The flower you're pressing isn't going to get better if you squish it unless you start with something that's good."

Do a test run
"A lot of different variables, like how long you press the bud down for, and what temperature the heating plates are, can drive the texture of the rosin that comes out. So when you get a new batch, test one gram or bud at a time, and see how it comes out at different temperatures."

Not all strains are created equal
"If you raise the temperature, the oils will come out runnier. So the right temperature and timing varies a lot from strain to strain. For example, Sour Tangie, which really does smell like tangerines, has a lot of essential oils and always comes out runny. Other strains come out almost solid as soon as the rosin cools, almost like taffy. This has to do with how rich in terpenes and oily that particular plant is."

Outdoor-grown weed is better
"Indoor and outdoor batches will also look totally different when you press them. A lot of indoor material looks really nice but might not have a super-high yield. Outdoor plants tend to have had more time to cultivate all their essential oils and terpenes out in the sun, so the rosin is usually very oily."

Freeze it
"If you're making edibles, it doesn't matter so much if the rosin is runny. But if you're dabbing, pop it in the freezer for a bit so that it's easier to work with and you don't have to fuss around with picking it off the parchment. After thirty seconds, it firms up enough that you can weigh out whatever amount you need."

Cook with concentrates
"The nice thing about cooking with rosin—or concentrates in general—is that once you've tested it, you know the potency, and you only have to use a very, very small amount. You don't have to deal with doing an infusion [steeping weed in liquid], then straining out plant material and wasting some of it; you get 100 percent yield. You can just weigh out the tiny bit that you need for your batch, and it melts right in and distributes really beautifully, as opposed to if you had to add weed butter or something else."

Get tested
"It's important to know that your edibles are consistent and that everyone knows what they're getting. Use a home cannabis testing kit like tCheck, which measures THC and other cannabinoid potency. Or, if you're lucky enough to be somewhere like California, you can buy product that's already been tested. Some labs also offer testing, so you can take a sample in. Dosage is very, very crucial."

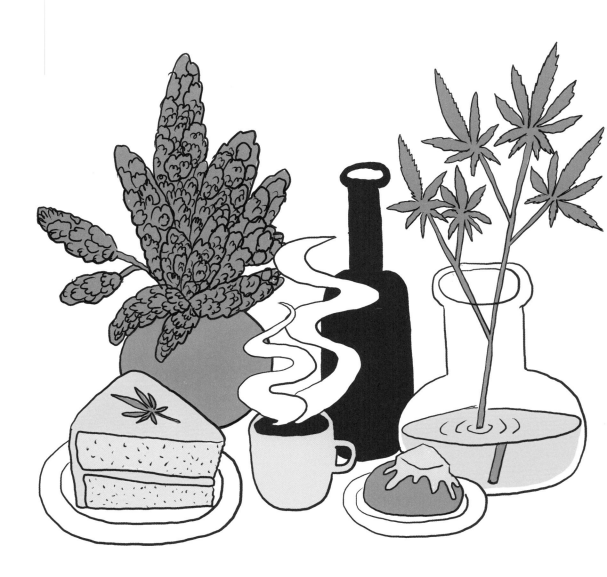

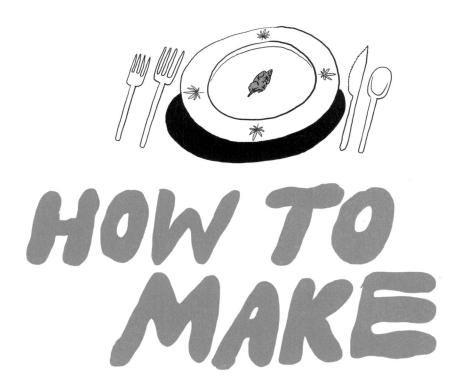

HOW TO MAKE

Congratulations, you've figured out how to smoke weed. Now it's time to eat it, drink it, and rub it all over your body.

There's a myriad of ways to mess around with weed in the kitchen. Since nothing's better than giving in to total stoner indulgence, we're starting with classic recipes for *baked* goods—best paired with pillow forts and hours of reality TV. Save these for your laziest days.

On the other hand, getting so high you can't feel your face isn't always helpful when you've got things to do. Luckily, the new wave of weed culture is all about health over hedonism. Which is why we've included a handy primer to microdosing—and packed in some healthy recipes for when you're hitting the gym or office and need a little boost.

Finally, for the nights you're in the mood for love, seduce your date with a *high*-end meal stolen straight from the kitchen of LA's favorite weed chef. If you get lucky, maybe the section on lotions and lube will come in handy.

We've come a long way from the pot brownie, baby.

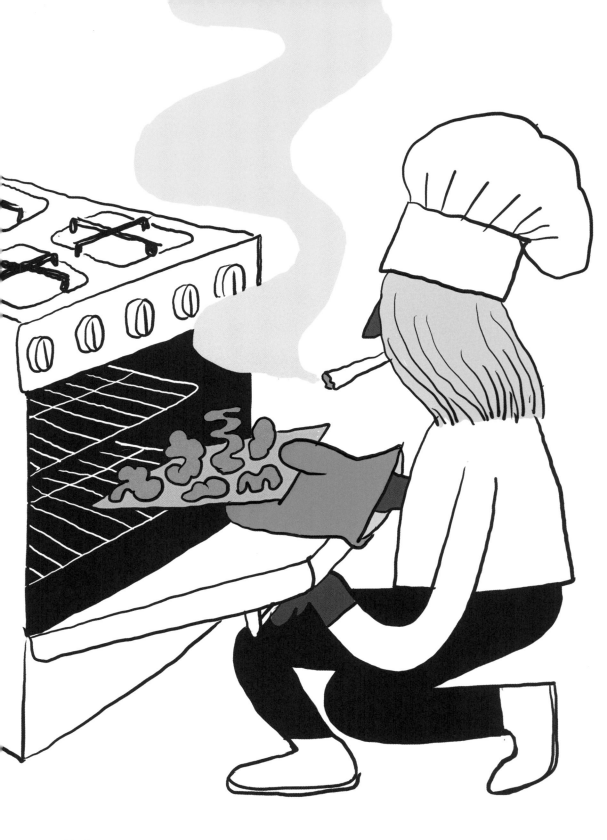

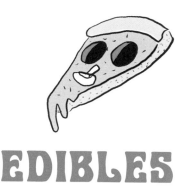

EDIBLES

Think of any kind of food—anything in the world—and someone's figured out a way to put weed in it. And why not? Edibles get you buzzed without harshing your lungs with smoke—*and* they taste delicious. It's hardly surprising that this corner of the cannabis universe is exploding.

Still, edibles have a pretty bad rep—freakouts are practically a hazing ritual to join the Real Stoners Club. You've probably heard horror stories of edible-induced meltdowns, if you haven't had one yourself. The thing is, most bad trips boil down to a simple root cause: you ate too much, fool! Which is why most edible experiences go like this: "I don't feel anything … I still don't feel anything … I'm sooo sober … ohmygodI'MDYINGCALLMYMOM!!!"

I'm going to tell you a secret: if you know your numbers (counting your intake by the milligram and paying attention to the time), you have nothing to fear. To help you with that, we're

kicking off this section with a dosage guide and other sciencey stats you should immediately imprint on your brain.

While many cannabis snacks aim to give you max potency for your buck, nibbling on a weed cookie while worrying you're going to black out isn't your only option. Low-dose edibles are also on the upswing, especially at cannabis dinners where you chow down multiple courses of weed-laced food. (Of course, there's still a cumulative effect— I once went to a weed dinner and stand-up comedy show where the last act was so baked that he just sat on stage for ten minutes, silently eating dessert with his eyes shut. It was the funniest performance of the night.)

So let's dig in. Here are some recipes for making your own weed treats, from sweet potato pecan cannabis cake bites to chia seed pudding, plus some pro tips from some of the coolest weed chefs out there.

How to Decarb Weed

Eating raw weed won't get you high, but it will leave you with an awful grassy taste in your mouth and a sinking sense that you just did something really dumb. This is because weed needs to be "decarboxylated" (that's a fancy way of saying "heated up") in order for it to actually produce any effects. So every time you cook with weed, always make sure it is "decarbed" first by following these steps:

1. Grind your cannabis.
2. Spread it thinly over a sheet of parchment paper on a baking sheet.
3. Set the oven to 220–235°F (100–110°C).
4. Bake for 30 to 45 minutes—and voilà, your weed is ready to get *you* baked.

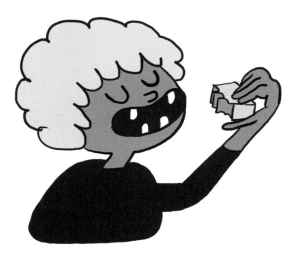

Weed Butter

An all-time classic. Spread over toast, pour over popcorn, or use it to make desserts.

What you'll need:
Weed
Butter

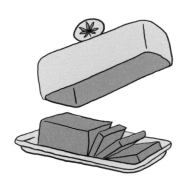

First, decarb your weed.

Add an equal amount of water and butter (e.g. 1 cup of each) to a pan. Bring to a simmer over low heat. As the butter melts, add your pot. Let the mixture simmer, covered, for 2 to 3 hours, stirring occasionally. Don't let it boil or burn. (You can also do this in a crockpot or slow cooker, in which case there's no need to add any water.)

Remove from the heat and let the butter cool, then strain out the weed by pouring it through cheesecloth into a container. The butter will keep for a few weeks in the refrigerator and up to six months in the freezer.

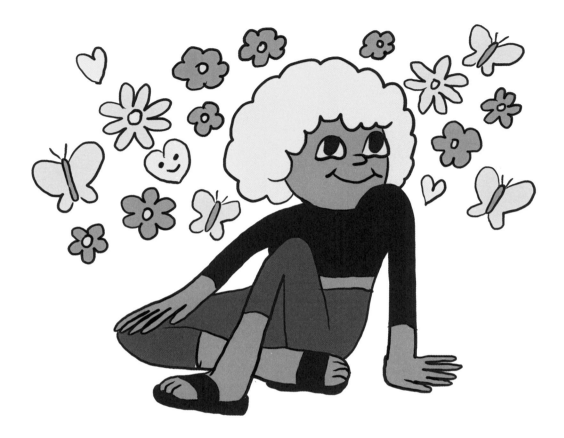

Edibles Dosage Guide

One thing best not learned the hard way: you cannot die from consuming too much weed, even if you're lying on the ground sweating and swearing that you will. Eating weed can be a completely different experience from smoking it—sometimes it almost seems like another drug entirely. (In fact, it kind of is. With edibles, THC becomes 11-Hydroxy-THC after passing through the stomach and liver. With smoking, it enters the bloodstream directly as delta-9-THC. These different chemical structures for THC will have different effects.)

Many people have intense, psychedelic trips after taking too big a bite of a weed brownie, and even the most hardcore stoner probably has an edible-induced horror story or two. Everyone responds to THC differently: some people flip out on low dosages, while others plow through high doses like tanks. Which is why it's crucial to know how much you're taking; if you're ever in doubt, just microdose (see p. 82).

THC Levels
Newbie: 2.5 to 5 mg
Standard: 5 to 10 mg (10 mg is considered
                    a single dose)
Stoner: 10 to 50 mg
Hardcore: 50+ mg

Note: Sometimes product labels will include a ratio like "1:1 THC:CBD."

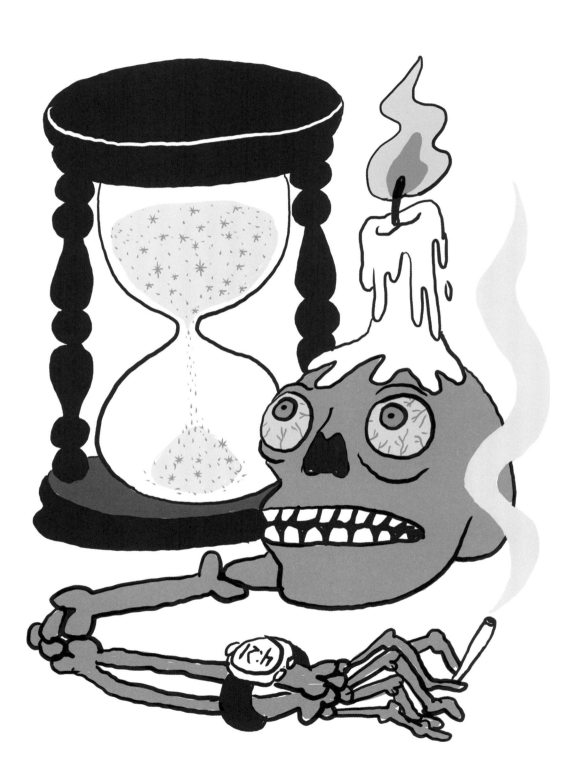

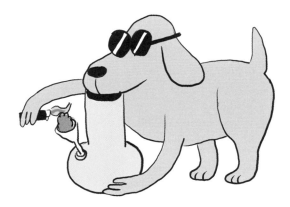

Average High Time Spans

Aside from dosage, *how* you ingest weed is the most important factor determining the time span of your high. The effects from smoking hit you fastest—usually within seconds—because they enter your system through your lungs and directly through your blood–brain barrier. THC from edibles is absorbed through your stomach, and it can take an hour or more for the effects to creep up. Infused drinks and tinctures, which seep in sublingually, are somewhere in the middle; you'll feel their effects within five to thirty minutes.

Of course, all of this also varies based on experience. Your body builds a tolerance to THC, so the more you smoke, the shorter the highs. Still, it's helpful to have a rough sense of how long you'll be stoned—just in case, you know, you have "real life" to take care of later.

Smoking
Feel effects in 5 minutes
Peak in 30 minutes
Lasts 2 to 4 hours total

Edibles
Feel effects in 40 to 90 minutes
Peak lasts for 3 to 4 hours
Lasts 5 to 10 hours total

Drinks
Feel effects in 30 minutes or less
Peak at 90 minutes
Lasts 2 to 4 hours total

Tinctures
Feel effects in 15 to 45 minutes
Peak at 90 minutes
Lasts 2 to 4 hours total

HIGH DINING
WITH CHEF LUKE REYES

A dimly lit restaurant with shiny black walls and red lanterns sits on a West Hollywood boulevard lined with streetwear and shoe stores. If it wasn't for the sharp smell of oil and Chinese food in the air, you might confuse it for a nightclub. Past a beaded curtain, in a kitchen clamoring with metal trays and orders shouted in Spanish and Mandarin, chef Luke Reyes is standing at a table in the corner, making dozens of weed dumplings.

Reyes runs La Hoja, a roving cannabis dining series that kicked off in late 2017. Tonight, he's preparing a five-course infused dinner, serving up spicy chicken wings, fried rice, and other Chinese American foods that late-night stoner dreams are made of. As his tattooed arms scoop creamy cheese infused with weed peanut oil into the flour dumpling wraps, Reyes speaks about his journey as a cannabis chef, wiping sweat off his brows and enthusiastically cursing with every other word.

How did you become a cannabis chef?
I grew up on the East Coast surrounded by people in the cannabis industry—honestly, I sold weed from my mid-teens into my early twenties. Then I started working in a bunch of James Beard Award-winning kitchens and the Four Seasons hotel in New York, and cooking became my livelihood. When I moved to Los Angeles in 2010, weed was still illegal, but I had friends who were growing and dealing it. They would come back from trimming [on weed farms] up north and be like, "Here's two pounds—can you do anything with it?" And I would throw it in my freezer and mess with it.

Then, about a year ago, I randomly got hit up by a casting director for a [competitive cannabis cooking] show called Cooking On High. I did the show and won a couple episodes. Not being a cunt, but a lot of people on the show were not real chefs. They were like, guys and girls who go to Burning Man every year and make brownies for friends, but don't know how to cook a piece of fish. So the entrepreneur side of me was like, if these guys are doing dinners and making money, why can't I do dinners with my friends in the cannabis industry, and make food that's actually good?

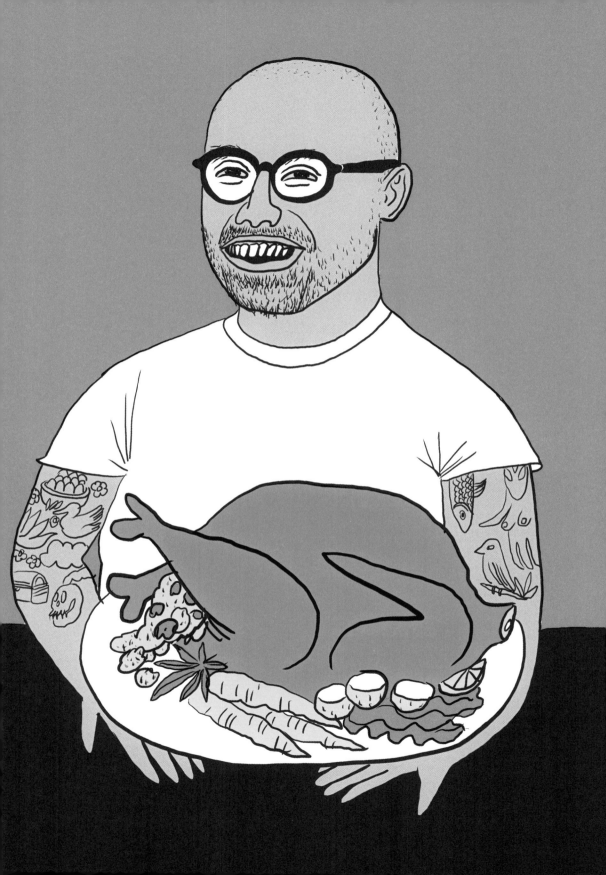

There seems to be a new school of cannabis cooking that's more about the food itself, as opposed to just getting blasted.

Usually when you talk to someone about edibles, they're like, "Oh shit, I had the worst experience …" I looked at some products at dispensaries, but it's like 200 mg of THC for three slices of pizza. You can't enjoy that because you're on the moon. Tonight, our dinner will be 30 mg. I'm using a bottle of THC-infused peanut oil to measure it all out—each dish has one tablespoon containing 5 mg. It's not so much about the high—we want people to enjoy the food.

Most edible recipes require weed oil or butter. Do you find this to be limiting?

Not at all! There are home infusers that allow you to do a lot of things, so you don't have to always start with a fat. We work with a company called CO_2 Clear, who are good friends of mine. We met through the first dinner I ever did, in a kinda sketchy warehouse we rented in downtown LA. So every time we do a dinner, I'll create a menu with them. They have a proprietary fusion technique they've mastered over the last ten years, and we can do soy sauce, sake, peanut oil … they've opened up what we can do.

Have you discovered new culinary possibilities through cooking with weed?

Cooking with weed is about more than just the flavor profile. You're also playing with the "high" profile. For example, you want to infuse the first course with a sativa strain that gets you high and bright. I'm working with a bunch of different strains with different terpenes. If you look at weed as more than just the psychoactive component, the possibilities are endless.

How does being a person of color affect your approach to the cannabis space?

I'm Puerto Rican-Irish, and my entire family— my older brothers and father—have been incarcerated because of cannabis. What's really important for me about cannabis is the social justice side for minorities who are unfairly targeted—it's much more likely that a seventeen-year-old black teenager will go to jail for a dimebag than a kid from the suburbs. With legalization, revisiting those cases is one of the most important things. Maybe we can't right those wrongs, but at least we can take a harder look at how we treat our youth and minorities.

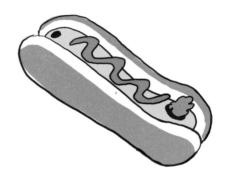

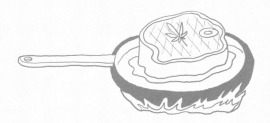

Pro Tips from Chef Reyes

Taste first, infuse later

"In a non-cannabis kitchen, you're continuously tasting and re-tasting things as you cook. But if you do that in an infused kitchen, you're nibbling a chicken wing, tasting your salad dressing, and all of a sudden you're super-high. So now, I'll do a batch of sauce, taste it before I cook, and add the infused distillate later."

Watch out for potency if you're using heat

"Sometimes, heating up an infused substance can increase its THC potency, because you're essentially decarbing the weed twice. So that's something to be careful of. For example, when we infuse sesame oil, if we bring it over 350 degrees, it slightly increases the THC content. So when we use it for fried rice or noodles, instead of 5 mg, we use 2.5 mg."

Go for top-shelf weed instead of leftover, lower-quality shake

"When I first started cooking in kitchens, I was using a cheap wine from Trader Joe's called Two-Buck Chuck to braise short ribs, but chefs in fine dining restaurants would use $10 to $12 bottles of wine. I'd be like, 'you're just deglazing!', but they made me realize that wine is an ingredient too, so why use cheap wine on thirty-day dry-aged short ribs? The better the starting ingredient, the better the end product—and that applies to weed, too."

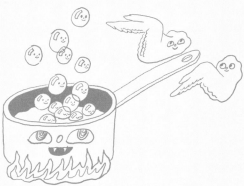

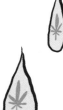

Chef Reyes's Cannabis-Infused Olive Oil

What you'll need:
3½ cups (840 ml) virgin olive oil
1 oz. (28 g) marijuana, finely ground
Coffee grinder
Cheesecloth
Lidded jar

Use a coffee grinder to get the marijuana as powdery as possible. Usually you can fit about 7 grams in these little grinders at a time, and they do a very good job of giving you a fine powder.

Start by putting the oil in a saucepan and warming it over medium heat. Don't let the oil reach its boiling point, but once it has heated up you can add in the marijuana powder.

Let the oil simmer, never letting it boil, stirring constantly. If you see bubbles begin to form in the oil, turn down the heat and remove the pan from the burner until it cools off a bit. By boiling the mixture, too much THC will be released and you won't get the desired effect from your oil.

Continue this for about an hour, possibly two if you have the time.

Strain the oil through cheesecloth into a jar or other container that you can cap. Be careful to let the oil cool a bit before doing this, as it'll be extremely hot right off the stove. Also, make sure to squeeze the cheesecloth at the end so you get all the oil out of it. Store in a jar.

You now have your marijuana-infused cannabis oil!

Chef Reyes's Herb-Roasted Chicken with Cannabis Lemon Vinaigrette

What you'll need:
1 whole chicken
2 cups (480 ml) THC-infused olive oil
2 lemons, zested and juiced
4 shallots, peeled and julienned
1 cup (240 ml) extra virgin olive oil
Dried chili flakes
3 avocados
A large bunch of sorrel, roughly chopped
1 small bag mixed lettuce
1 cup feta cheese, crumbled
1 bunch thyme
1 bunch rosemary
Kosher salt
Black pepper
Kitchen twine

Using a pastry brush, spread some of the infused olive oil over the entire chicken, then rub or pat kosher salt and black pepper onto the breast, legs, and thighs. Place the chicken in a large resealable plastic bag. Set the open bag in a large bowl, keeping the chicken breast side up. Chill in the refrigerator for at least 8 hours and up to 2 days.

Arrange a rack in the upper third of your oven; preheat it to 500°F (260°C). Set a wire rack in a large heavy roasting pan. Remove the chicken from the bag. Pat it dry with paper towels (do not rinse it). Place the chicken breast side up on the pan rack and place half the thyme and half the rosemary inside the cavity. Loosely tie the legs together with kitchen twine and tuck the wing tips under. Brush the chicken all over with some of the infused oil and scatter the remaining herbs over the top.

Roast the chicken, brushing again with the infused olive oil after 15 minutes, until the skin is light-golden-brown and taut—about 30 minutes. Reduce the oven temperature to 350°F (175°C). Remove the chicken from the oven and brush with more oil. Leave it to rest for 15 to 20 minutes.

While the chicken is resting, pour 1 cup (240 ml) of infused olive oil into a chilled bowl, and add the lemon juice and zest along with the julienned shallots, whisking in 2 tbsp chili flakes, 1 cup extra virgin olive oil, and kosher salt to taste.

Cut the avocados in half, discarding the pits, and scoop the flesh out. Cut the flesh into ½-inch (1.5-cm) cubes and place in the bowl with the lemon dressing. Add the sorrel and lettuces and mix lightly.

Return the chicken to the oven and roast until the skin is golden-brown and a thermometer inserted into the thickest part of the thigh registers 165°F (75°C); about 40 to 45 minutes. Remove it from the oven, let it rest for 20 minutes, then carve.

Place the dressed avocado and greens onto a plate and put the carved chicken on top. Sprinkle the feta over the chicken and salad, and lightly spoon any leftover dressing onto the chicken.

Q&A

WEED FOR WELLNESS WITH MOONMAN'S MISTRESS

What happens when a nutritionist and a personal trainer start a weed company? An edibles empire that makes paleo-friendly vegan cookies, and throws boot camps on the side. San Francisco's MoonMan's Mistress, co-founded by Liz Rudner and Jamel Ramiro, is part of the new "healthy pothead" wave sweeping modern weed culture. Their THC- and CBD-rich cookies—which have won awards from big-deal festivals like the Emerald Cup—are made for stoners who'd rather hit a CrossFit gym or hot yoga class than melt into their couch. The company also throws boot-camp-style fitness classes where, at the end of a grueling hour, you're rewarded with a bag of CBD edibles and lotions to help with muscle recovery. Here, Rudner shares some thoughts on cannabis and exercise—including how everyone wants to open a weed gym. Don't miss her recipe for cake bites, either.

How would you define the lazy stoner stereotype?
The "lazy stoner" is thought to be inactive and irresponsible—a couch potato always having the munchies for junk food. Someone who is as unhealthy as it gets. The cannabis space is working really hard to change this stigma as it charges head-first into the mainstream.

How are you trying to move away from this cliché?
MoonMan's Mistress has always catered to the active person's lifestyle. Jamel, my business partner, is a master trainer, and I am a holistic nutritionist. Our company embodies the wellness lifestyle not just by stamping the word "healthy" on our packaging; we also sponsor high-performing athletes, partner with Ganja Yoga [a cannabis-enhanced yoga class], and host Burn & Baked fitness events. And we participate in wellness-centered events throughout San Francisco, from

brunches to pop-up dinners, wellness gatherings to sound healing.

What is the goal of your Burn & Baked boot camp?
The goal of Burn & Baked is to dismantle the "lazy stoner" stereotype, and share with the world that people from all walks of life can benefit from cannabis, notably CBD. If you eat well, you'll move well. If you can move well, you'll sleep well. This trifecta is the key to living well!

Speaking of cannabis and exercise, what do you think about weed gyms?
At first, everyone was going a bit crazy in California talking about opening cannabis gyms. But the reality is that the cannabis industry has a long way to go before the general population is okay with the idea of cannabis usage, let alone cannabis and wellness in the same industry. Maybe when the insurance and banking industries stop being blockers, a stand-alone cannabis gym will be possible. As a small brand, we're just hopeful that the new laws allow for small, health-conscious products to stay on the market and grow with this ever-changing landscape.

What are the best ways to incorporate weed into an active lifestyle?
I don't think there's a specific formula because everyone's body metabolizes weed differently. For example, Jamel is a high-performing athlete and is more of a nighttime user who focuses on the anti-inflammatory benefits of CBD. His daytime use is primarily only on big surf days when he wants to calm his anxiety. On the other hand, I'm a balanced daytime and nighttime user and my consumption is much greater. Consuming THC before a workout, especially for my yoga practice, allows me to perform and focus better through each movement.

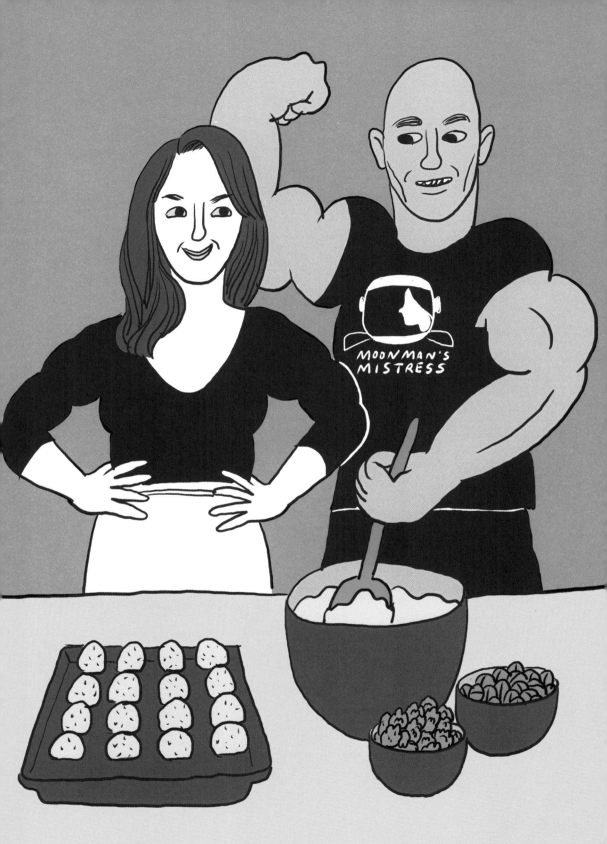

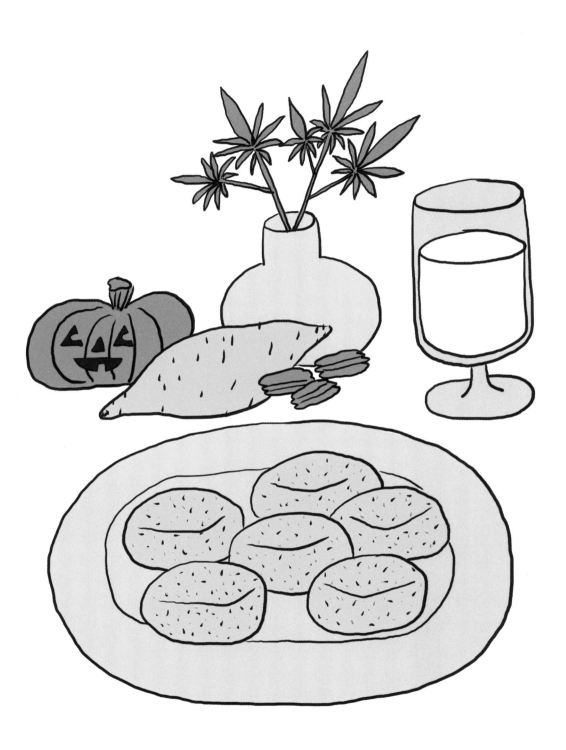

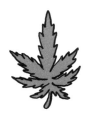

MoonMan's Mistress's Sweet Potato Pecan Cannabis Cake Bites

(Gluten-free, vegan, low-GI)

What you'll need:
3 cups almond flour
½ cup shredded coconut
¼ cup flax meal
2 tbsp coconut flour
1 tbsp pumpkin pie spice
½ tsp baking soda
½ tsp baking powder
½ tsp salt
½ cup sweet potato puree
½ cup maple syrup
½ cup organic cannacoconut oil
1 tbsp pure vanilla extract
½ cup chopped raw pecans

Preheat the oven to 325°F (160°C).

In a large mixing bowl, combine the dry ingredients (except the pecans).

In a small mixing bowl, combine the sweet potato puree, maple syrup, melted cannacoconut oil and vanilla extract with a hand mixer.

Stir the wet ingredients into the dry ingredients. Once everything is mixed together, add the chopped pecans and stir through.

Drop tablespoon-sized amounts of batter onto a parchment-lined baking sheet. Bake for 15 to 18 minutes, until the bottoms are lightly browned. Allow the cake bites to cool before serving.

MICRODOSING WITH EMILY O'BRIEN OF MONDO

Recently, microdosing has gone from a Silicon Valley trend touted by tech bros to an increasingly mainstream phenomenon popular with everyone from soccer moms to magazine editors. The idea is simple: instead of popping a full edible or smoking a whole joint, you take small, incremental doses of cannabis in order to enjoy its benefits without getting messed up. It's the perfect way to go if you're using weed to work and want to be productive instead of melting into your couch or floating in some tripped-out mental headspace.

Emily O'Brien is the one-woman powerhouse behind Mondo, a cannabis powder made specifically for microdosing. Each jar comes with a precise 5 mg scoop—what Emily calls a "minimal effective dose" designed to help people get clarity without losing focus.

When we met at a comedy show hosted by a high-end edibles company, O'Brien was standing at her booth behind jars of Mondo powder. With her cropped blonde hair and wicked smile, she exuded an air of confidence and spoke at a fast clip as she rattled off the many mental and physical benefits of microdosing.

Why is microdosing good for you?
The whole concept of microdosing is about allowing the body to get back into a state of balance, and the beautiful thing about it is that you don't have to do it every day. Cannabis, like alcohol, is biphasic, which means that it's really good up to a certain point, and then it's really negative. So everyone can benefit from microdosing 1 or 2 mg of THC, but not everyone can benefit from, you know, 10, 15, or 20 mg.

Microdosing can be done every single day, regardless of time of day. Taking such a small amount is just enough to make you breathe a little bit easier and be a little bit more open, but not enough to have any sort of psychoactive effect. The point is to rebalance the body, including reducing inflammation, helping your immune system calm down from allergies, and mental clarity.

How exactly does it work?
I find that microdosing through edibles is the best way, because it has the longest activation time. Once you know your dosage, whether it's 2 mg or 5 mg, put on a timer and wait to feel it out.

Cannabis powders like Mondo are one of the best ways to microdose, because it gets into your system faster and hits you like a joint would. The THC is bound by tapioca starch, a simple carbohydrate that our saliva can easily break down. So when it hits your tongue, it dissolves instantaneously, and the THC has a huge surface area with which to be absorbed.

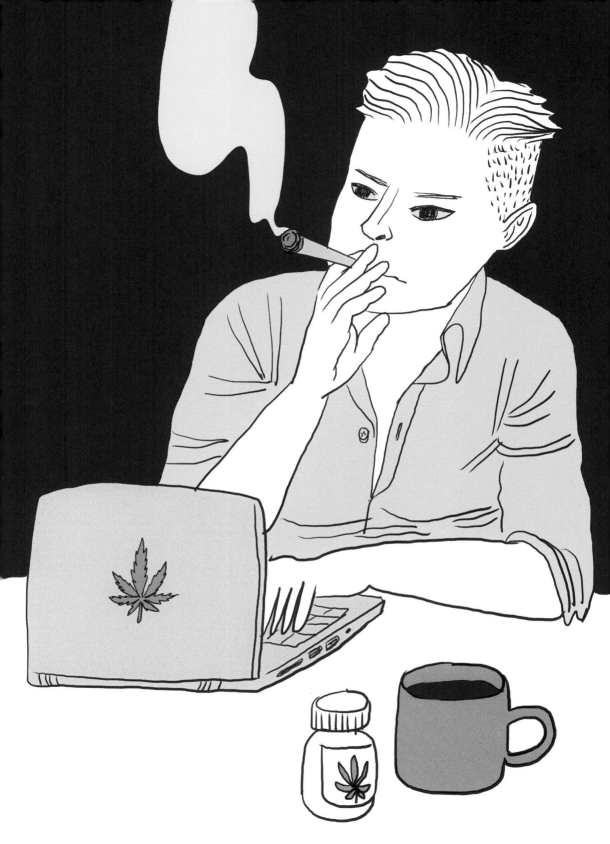

If someone is trying to decide what the best way to microdose is for them, would you recommend different methods depending on what they're looking for?

Yes, I would! If you're looking for mental clarity I would recommend delta-9-THC ingestion. So that could be eating a cannabis powder like Mondo, or it could be using a vape pen like Dosist, where each puff is 2 mg. If you're smoking, you have to do it every 90 minutes, because it's only active for a short amount of time. If you're microdosing for more body-oriented stuff, like reducing your blood pressure or itchy allergies, edibles are a great way to go. I would recommend very precision-controlled edibles like mints, or anything else small-scale.

Can you explain what delta-9-THC is?

When you're growing cannabis, what's growing on the flower is THCA, which is non-psychoactive. If you were to get cannabis leaves and juice them, it wouldn't get you high, but THCA is really beneficial for inflammation, helping children with ADHD, and things like that. As soon as you harvest the flower, roll it up into a joint, and smoke it, it goes from THCA to delta-9-THC, and that's the psychoactive part that gets you stoned.

When you're eating cannabis, it's digested in your stomach and goes into your liver, and it changes from delta-9-THC into 11-hydroxy-THC, which is a whole different high. It's much more body-heavy. Also, sometimes with edibles you can really tell what kind of strain it is, whether it's a sativa or indica.

What's the best strain for microdosing?

I've found that 2 mg of Blue Dream is the most effective for a daytime anti-anxiety dose. The reason being that 2 mg of THC is just enough for you to feel like, "Oh okay, I kind of feel something working," but it's not enough to be stoned. And the Blue Dream plant is beneficial because it has a wonderful combination of terpenes. Most present in Blue Dream is beta-caryophyllene—this super-chill terpene also found in black peppercorns that makes everything just feel better. It also has a one-to-one ratio of the sativa terpene pinene and the indica terpene myrcene, so essentially it's a calm, euphoric, anxiety-relieving combination of terpenes.

Are the benefits of microdosing backed up by stats and science?

There was a wonderful study done showing how microdosing in older life really helps with memory recall—so it has bigger benefits for older people. This study showed that younger mice did super-well at the beginning of the [memory] test, and older mice did as expected. After four weeks of microdosing THC, the older mice outperformed the younger mice in the first round, and they saw the same results for the next six weeks. When they stopped giving them THC, [the researchers] saw that the mice's brains were still processing as if they still had THC in their system.

The US has a patent on cannabis that actually says that it's a neuroprotectant and can help prevent Alzheimer's and Parkinson's disease. So this study backs that up. This is also really cool because THC could help people replace their pharmaceutical medication with ones that aren't as addictive.

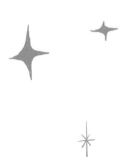

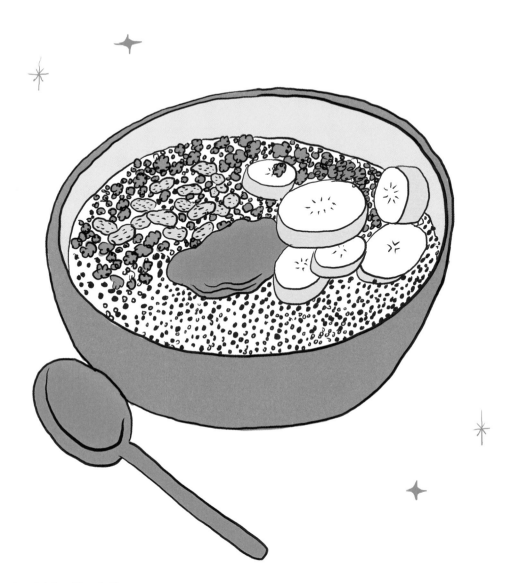

Mondo's Chia Pudding

What you'll need:
¾ can light coconut milk
¼ cup (60 ml) almond milk (or milk of choice)
½ cup chia seeds
¼ cup maple syrup
Splash of vanilla extract (approx. ½ tsp)
Pinch Himalayan salt
2 to 4 scoops cannabis powder
Toppings of your choice, to serve

Toss everything into a bowl and mix together. Let sit, refrigerated, overnight or for at least 2 hours.

Serve topped with blueberries, raspberries, or golden raisins. For a more tropical flavor, include cut mangos, bananas, or crushed pineapple; for a summer vibe, go with strawberry coulis, blueberries, or edible flowers. If you'd like it to be more filling, add bananas, a swirl of peanut butter, cacao nibs, or shredded coconut.

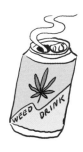

DRINKS

Weed drinks have long been considered odd ducks in the edibles world. But in recent years their popularity has started to take off, thanks to the collective realization that drinking cannabis gets you stoned faster than eating it does, so you don't have to sit around waiting for an hour or longer for the effects to kick in.

Most weed drinks, especially the ones sold at legal dispensaries, don't contain alcohol. This is because alcohol and weed risks the dreaded cross-fade feeling—when you start to get the spins and feel sick, or just uncomfortable.

Research suggests that there are ways to get around this, though. According to several studies, if you smoke first, then drink alcohol, the weed in your system actually causes blood alcohol levels to be lower than if you'd only drunk alcohol. But if you do it the other way around—drink first, then smoke—the alcohol has the opposite effect on the THC, causing you to get more stoned than usual. (This happens because alcohol opens up your blood vessels, helping more THC get absorbed.) Since, realistically, you're probably going to be doing both at the same time, just be careful and go slow.

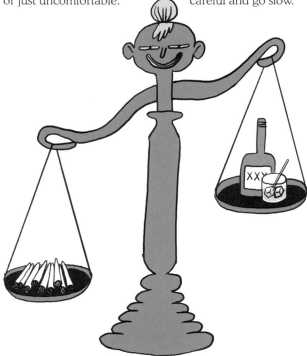

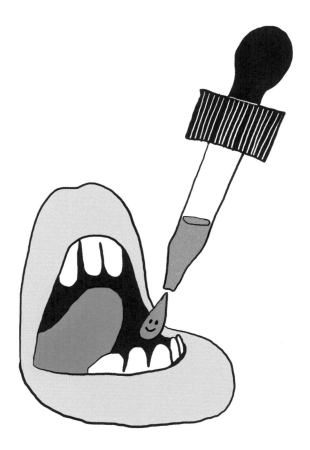

Weed Tincture

Unlike edibles, weed tinctures are great because they don't expire or get gross and moldy. They can also be a more health-conscious alternative to high-fat desserts. Start with 1 milliliter, and increase until you get to your perfect dose. To take it straight, drop the tincture under your tongue and hold it there for 30 seconds. Or add a healthy squirt to juices, smoothies, soups, or sauces to get stoned off your next meal.

What you'll need:
1 oz. (28 g) decarbed weed (see p. 68)
1 pint (approx. 500 ml) of the highest-proof
  alcohol you can get (such as Everclear)
Resealable bag
Mason jar
Coffee filter
Flavored extracts such as vanilla (optional)
Large, dark-tinted tincture bottle with dropper

Put your decarbed weed into a resealable bag and pop both the pot and the alcohol into the freezer. Leave them there for a couple hours.

Once the buds are frozen, grind them up almost into a powder (using your fingers or a grinder), and mix with the alcohol in a Mason jar.

Close the jar and shake it vigorously for at least five minutes, then put it back into the freezer. Leave it there for at least 48 hours, giving the jar a shake every few hours.

Strain the liquid through a coffee filter into another jar or a bowl, to remove any remaining particles. If you want the tincture to be extra tasty, add a flavored extract like vanilla.

Transfer the tincture to a dark or opaque bottle. Stored away from light it will keep indefinitely.

Cold-Busting Weed Elixir

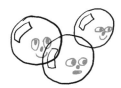

This soothing blend of honey, ginger, citrus, and weed tincture is the perfect remedy for cold nights, sore throats, or any time you just want to give your body a break.

What you'll need:
3 tbsp honey
½ oz. (14 g) decarbed weed (see p. 68)
3 oz. (85 ml) vodka
1 tsp grated ginger
1 tsp orange zest

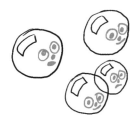

Heat the honey over low heat in a small saucepan, making sure not to let it foam.

Grind up your decarbed weed into a powder and stir it into the honey. Add the ginger and orange zest, then slowly add in the vodka.

Cook over a low heat. The mixture should stay liquid, not become a hot, sticky mess. After 30 minutes, pour into a jar and let it cool.

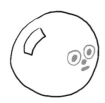

Take a teaspoon every 15 minutes, until you hit the right dose for you.

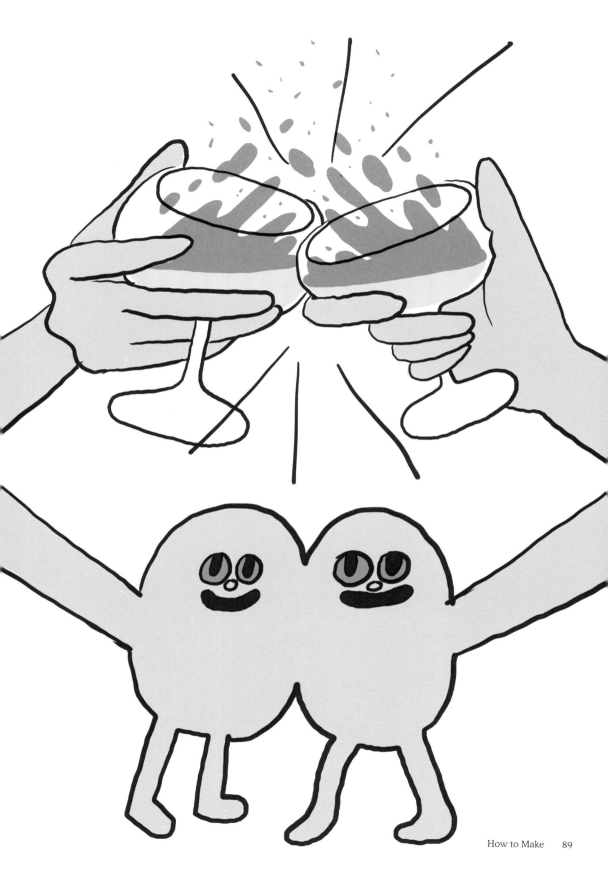

Q&A

WEED AND WINE WITH ALICIA ROSE OF HERBABUENA

Smoking and drinking at the same time can result in cross-fade—when you get the spins and have to hightail it out of the party before you throw up. But if you know what you're doing, mixing weed and alcohol can actually work to your advantage, elevating your senses and taste buds to create a rich gastronomic experience.

Alicia Rose worked in the wine industry for fifteen years before she started HerbaBuena, a California-based cannabis company with award-winning tinctures, edibles, and biodynamically grown flowers. In addition to selling cannabis products, HerbaBuena also hosts dinners where weed strains are carefully paired with different types of wine. With a foot in both worlds, Alicia wants to redefine the way we think about weed based on everything she's learned from the world of high-end vino.

Here, she elaborates on the fascinating cultural similarities between wine and weed—and how to combine them without getting too messed up.

What similarities do you see between weed and wine?
I've been working with extraordinary winemakers at the top of their game for close to twenty years. There are thousands of people who make it their life's work to be able to tell the difference between a right-bank or a left-bank Bordeaux variety, and other very esoteric but refined nuances of the sensual experience that is wine. It's not just a flavor, it's not just the smell—it's these incredible stories and the artists who created it. Cannabis does that too. Both wine and weed have the

ability to sort of transport you in this sensual, tactile, experiential kind of way.

How did you go from working in the wine industry to cannabis?
I love wine, the people in the industry, and living in wine country. It was a great way to marry my interest in agriculture with a more sophisticated, experiential consumer product and branding focus. At one point in my career, I could literally walk into a failing winery and have it turned around and profitable within three years. I got really good at it.

And yet whenever I was faced with the question, "Do you want to start your own wine brand?" or, "Are you interested in having a winery?", it just never felt like the passion that I wanted to live. When you hit a certain age, you start asking: what is my legacy? And for me it was really about having a platform to talk about the healing of people and the planet—and cannabis transcends wine in almost every way when you're coming at it from that perspective.

Wine takes us away from our worldly woes by almost separating us from them, right? We check out when we drink alcohol. Although the experience of drinking great wine is very sensual and connected, and is always better when shared with people, the alcohol itself actually takes us further from our deeper selves and our spiritual selves. That's why we black out, that's why we have drunk, sloppy sex, that's why all these things happen when we drink. It frees our inhibitions and helps us check out of our reality for a while.

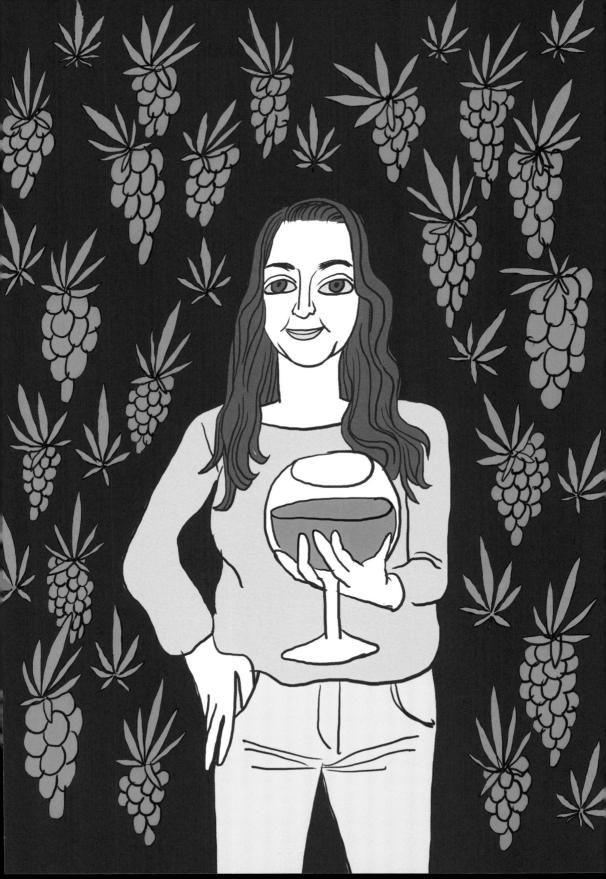

Cannabis, on the other hand, does the exact opposite. It is a therapeutic, healing plant that forces us to get more in tune with our spiritual, physical, and mental bodies. I believe that it has the ability to take you to a place of healing, giving, and nurturing, rather than extracting and checking out.

What parallels do you see between the artisan wine world and that of cannabis?
Both wine and cannabis are highly prized and highly regulated agricultural products that have the ability to often transform normal days into extraordinary ones. So when you think about it that way, the same attention and detail that goes into the cultivation, processing, bottling, and sale of a hundred-point wine for a world-class winery needs to go into the products that we are creating with cannabis.

Our longing to feel connected is something the wine industry has really capitalized on. We have these beautiful wineries where we bring people in and give them this very deep, tactile experience. We teach them how to taste it and experience it. We give them stories to take home and retell to their friends. It's how great wine brands were built. And the exact same thing has started to happen more with cannabis.

Do you think that legal cannabis could transform wine country? For example, I've heard that cannabis brands are taking over or pairing up with California wineries.
I believe that cannabis will have an extraordinary effect on wine culture—it's able to elevate the wine country experience by having people taste more but drink less. So they experience more, but check out less. At what we call "elevated epicurean experiences," we start out by telling people that cannabis is something that's actually going to allow you to experience wine or food more deeply and intimately. So instead of drinking three glasses of wine, you can take a hit of cannabis and then have a taste of your wine, and both things enhance each other.

If you ask any winery out there, their least favorite time of day is their 4 p.m. tasting because people show up and they're drunk. And you don't want to have to deal with drunk people when you're opening up $150 bottles of wine. It just goes to waste at that point. If people enjoy some cannabis and then go taste wine, they're actually enjoying the wine more and often have a better time because they're not hungover after.

There's this stoner mantra: "Bong before beer, you're in the clear—beer before grass, you're on your ass." We always make sure to tell people: You want to im*vibe*, which is to take your cannabis, before you im*bibe*, which is to drink. And the reason is that when you're drinking alcohol, the moment you become drunk, you check out in a way. So when you add THC to that, with the exponential effect of how THC and alcohol amplify each other, all of a sudden you're too impaired. When you have a little puff or a drop of tincture first, you're more in control of the high. You're more in control stoned than you are drunk.

Are there certain strains that work best for pairing with wine?
Absolutely. We usually start with the wine, and then we actually pair the cannabis to the wine. For example, you're going to want to pair a Petite Sirah—a big, meaty, dark-blue fruited wine—with something that has similar components, like musky berry- or cherry-flavored cannabis strains.

There are also different qualities of smoke, based not just on the strain but on the way a particular plant was grown and a particular phenotype. Often, the quality of great cannabis is not just looks—you know, super-green or with tons of crystals or super-tight nugs—but the quality of the smoke. The highest quality cannabis is, for me, a cannabis where the smoke has a creamy quality. Something that's very smooth and mouth-filling and round, just like a great wine. Hundred-point wines are balls of roundness in your mouth. You shouldn't feel anything sticking out, or any angles. The same thing goes for great cannabis. There should be nothing that's harsh or would make you cough or that lingers too long in your throat.

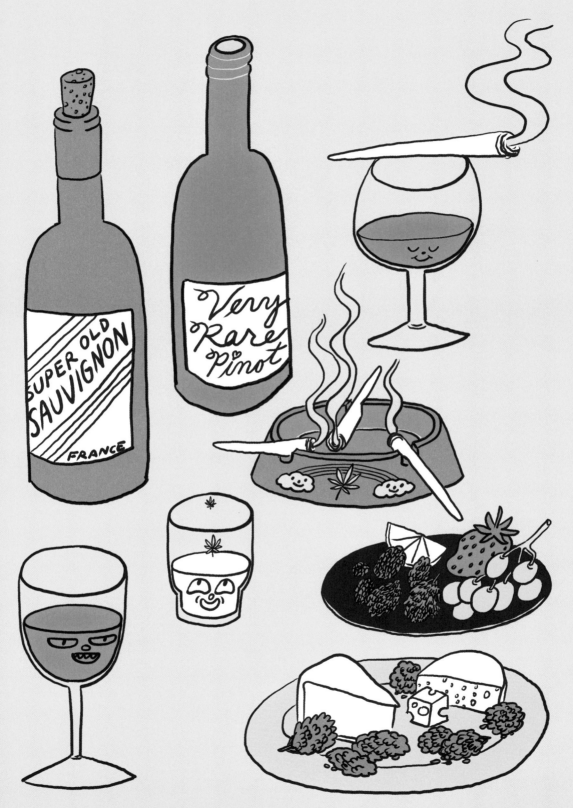

TOPICALS

"Topicals" refers to anything you can apply to your body, including lotions, salves, and creams. Because you're absorbing weed through your skin, you won't actually get stoned or experience any other mental effects—but it will provide relief from aches and pains, as well as other kinds of inflammation. Making topicals isn't too different from their edible counterparts. If you can make weed butter, you can make weed lotion with a couple extra steps.

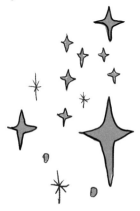

Weed Salve

What you'll need:
1½ cups (360 ml) coconut oil
10 g (⅓ oz.) decarbed weed (see p. 68)
½ cup (120 ml) beeswax
Your favorite essential oils (optional)
Cheesecloth
Lidded jar

Mix the coconut oil and weed in a saucepan over a very low heat, stirring constantly for 20 to 25 minutes. Remove from the heat and pour through a piece of cheesecloth into a jar. Set aside.

Slowly melt the beeswax in the saucepan, then add the infused coconut oil. Take it off the heat and put the mixture back into the jar.

Stir through a few drops of aromatherapeutic essential oils like lavender, peppermint, or tea tree. Allow to cool before putting the lid on.

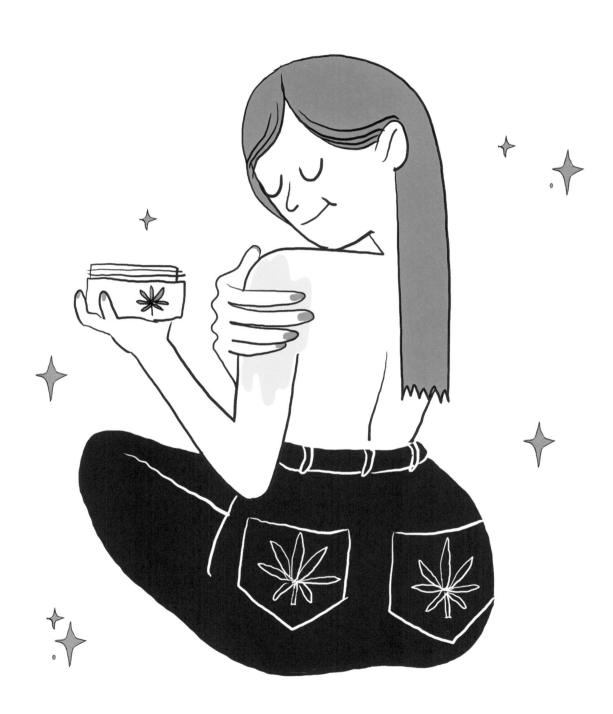

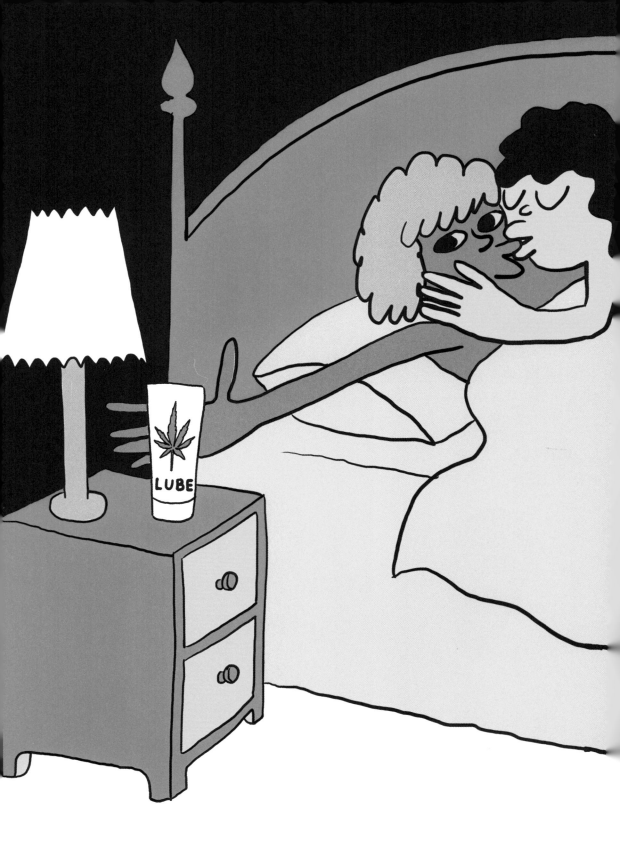

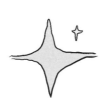
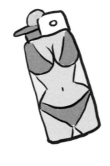

Weed and Sex

We've come to the part about weed and sex—also known as The Horny Section. If you're not into graphic discussions of dicks and vaginas, you might want to skip this part. But if you're like, "Stoned sex rules!" and want to learn more, read on.

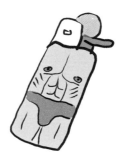

Weed Lube

Although it sounds like a joke, weed lube is actually a fun and surprisingly effective addition to the bedroom. THC dilates your capillaries to increase blood flow to even the smallest blood vessels in your body, thus enhancing sensitivity and sensation. All of which is to say: this actually works. And since lube is just a different way of saying "oil used in naughty ways," making your own is as easy as infusing a natural oil of your choice.

If you want to keep it simple
Go with coconut oil, which absorbs easily and contains lauric acid, a natural antimicrobial that helps to prevent infections.

If you have sensitive skin
Go with almond oil, which is light and rich in vitamin E.

If you're using latex condoms
Go with aloe vera oil, which is water-soluble. Other, fat-soluble oils can weaken latex condoms and cause them to break.

What you'll need:
6 cups (approx. 1.5 L) oil of your choice
1 oz. (28 g) ground-up, decarbed weed (see p. 68)
Airtight container

Slowly heat the oil in a saucepan over a low heat. Add your decarbed weed to the oil bit by bit, until it is completely mixed in. Simmer over low heat for 45 minutes, stirring occasionally.

Remove from the heat, let cool, and store in an airtight container. The lube will keep in the refrigerator for up to two months.

Q&A
STONED SEX
WITH ASHLEY MANTA

Combining weed and sex might sound like a dicey proposition. One puff too many and you've turned into a giggling slug rolling around the floor who's forgotten how your body parts work, much less how to mash them against another person. But the two can go together really well, if you know what you're doing.

Enter Ashley Manta, a sex educator who is the world's most famous "cannasexual." You can't mention weed and sex to someone in the industry without them bringing up Manta, who has dedicated her life to preaching the gospel of stoned sex. In addition to holding her own workshops, she is a regular speaker on the weed party scene, where she delivers her sex-positive message about embracing the benefits of cannabis in the bedroom.

And while the term "cannasexual" might sound like a bit of a stretch—try putting that on your Tinder bio and seeing how many eye rolls you get—Manta explains that it's more of a philosophy than a sexual orientation. When we meet one night in a Beverly Hills mansion at a VIP dinner for the California Cannabis Awards, Manta pulls me into a dimly lit back room. She smiles sweetly while reaching into her purse, pulling out a stuffed toy vagina, anatomically correct labia and all, to show me how to correctly apply weed lube. Then, tossing back her long blond hair, she proceeds to tell me all about the carnal uses of cannabis.

What's your definition of a "cannasexual"?
A cannasexual is anyone who mindfully and deliberately combines sex and cannabis to deepen intimacy and enhance pleasure. People think it's a sexual orientation, but it's not. Whether solo or partnered, canna-sexuality is meant to be a philosophy and a paradigm— a way of approaching sexuality with cannabis.

What does it mean to "meaningfully engage" with cannabis during sex?
I want people to be mindful of where they are pre-sex, where they want to be, and how cannabis can help them create the experience they're looking for.

If I come home after a long day of work and I'm feeling stressed out, maybe I have a headache, I want something with a high CBD content that's going to help me get out of my head and into my body. Or if I want to be sexy with my partner but my shoulder cramps up because I work on a computer all day, I can have my partner give me an infused massage.

I want people to think outside the box. It's not just about getting stoned and having sex. Anyone can do that. You don't have to be high to enjoy the benefits of cannabis during sex. There are topicals, there are high-CBD products. I'm really about the holistic approach in how to combine cannabis and sex.

How did you get started as a sex educator?
I've been a sex educator since right out of college, so I've been doing this for ten years. I got my start doing sexual violence protection and awareness as a rape crisis counselor and victim advocate. I worked at Planned Parenthood, so I got a really wide range of knowledge on sexuality.

The cannabis industry has only been around since 2014 or 2015, so I've been doing this for the last three and a half years. I realized there was a community of sex educators, therapists, bloggers, reviewers, and coaches, but there wasn't really anyone talking about cannabis and how to incorporate it in a mindful way—with an eye on consent and making sure everyone is safe and thrilled about being there.

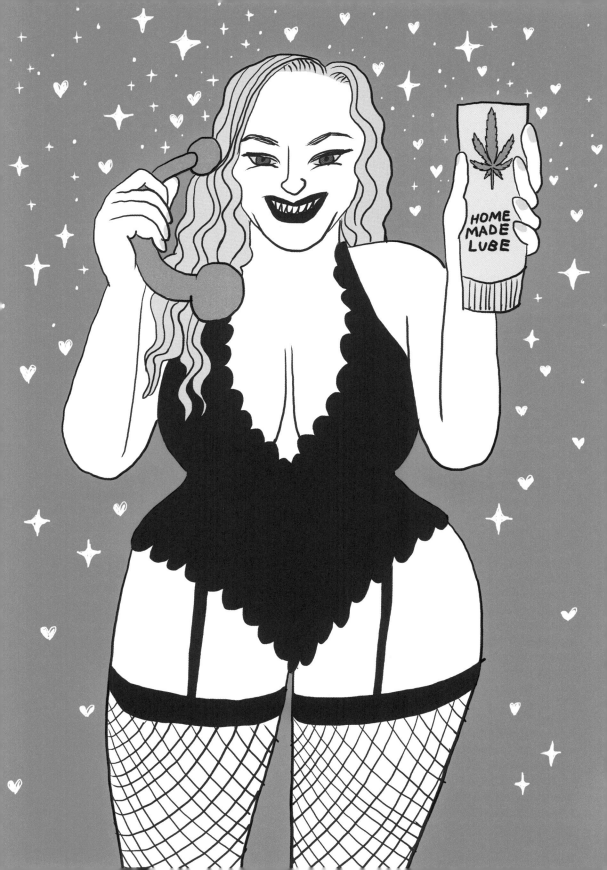

What do you think cannabis brings to the experience of sex?

It can do so many things. It can really help people get out of their head and into their body. It can increase pleasure, and decrease pain or discomfort.

What are some of the most creative ways you've incorporated cannabis into sex?

One of my colleagues came to me; she had been afraid to incorporate cannabis into her life but she was having back pain and it was keeping her from being present during sex. She was afraid of getting high and being sluggish. So I asked, "What if you were to dab CBD isolate?" It's flash-vaporizing something that is 99 percent CBD, so it's not going to get you "high." It's just going to completely relax your body and help with pain. So she did, and she and her partner went home and had amazing sex.

When did you start noticing that weed lube was "a thing"?

I first heard of weed lube in 2014. Foria was the first on the scene; it was a coconut-infused THC oil that you apply to your vulva. That was the first time I'd ever heard of a cannabis company specifically marketing their product toward sexual pleasure and reduction of pain, and that was revolutionary to me.

Weed lube became a phenomenon. The funny thing is, the name is very much a misnomer, because it's not like the lube you'd use during sex if you need more lubrication in the act. It's more of a marinade; you have to put it on 25 minutes before sexy-fun time begins and let it sit. I have people say, "We used it as lube and it didn't work," and I respond, "Yeah, you didn't let it sit long enough."

You can't use weed lube with latex condoms or they might break, right?

Right. Weed lube companies weren't doing a great job of educating about not using nitrile or polyurethane condoms early on, but they started to make it clearer over time. As more people started entering the weed lube phenomenon, the industry came out with a suppository.

How does weed lube work?

You spray it onto the mucosa, the wet part of the vagina. So it's not really about getting it on the outside lips or the mons pubis. It's about getting it inside the lips, right on the clit. Because the area's so open and absorbent, the THC goes straight into the tissue and then the nerves. THC is a vasodilator; it widens blood vessels, so more blood can go through. So when you have more blood flow in anything, it gets a little bit red and is more sensitive. There's more oxygen, more sensation; it's decreasing pain and increasing pleasure.

And then when you add CBD, you're adding more anti-inflammatory awesomeness. You can either do just THC or CBD, or both together—although I don't find the last to be as effective as CBD alone.

You don't get stoned right?

You don't, but if your partner goes down on you, your vagina is now an edible—at two and a half milligrams per spray. So if you put five sprays on there, that's not a small amount of THC that your partner just ingested.

Does weed lube work on penises?

I've had some people with a penis say it feels a little more sensitive, but for the most part, because of the way you have to spray weed lube on and let it sit, it wouldn't have the time to sink in. So the mechanism of absorption is not as effective.

Ashley Manta's Tips for Using Cannabis During Sex

Negotiate before you medicate

"Consent is vital and mandatory, especially if you're going to be using anything that has psychoactive effects. Have a conversation beforehand about what's on the table, including safe words and how to let someone know if you're not having a good time."

Microdosing is the move

"Cannabis, especially when it comes to sexuality, has a very steep cut-off point where it stops being fun and starts being lousy. There's a line, and everyone's line is in a slightly different place, so you have to find it, and you want to stay on the right side of that line. Once you go past it you're sleepy, you're lethargic, you're disconnected, and you might be paranoid. So figure out what you need and which strain or product is going to get you there. Then use the smallest amount you need to get the effects you're looking for."

What's the best strain for sex?

"It depends on what kind of sex you're trying to have; how much time you have; your favorite method of consumption; whether you want to be high; and where you'll be when you get started. The only reliable way to figure out how cannabis sex works best for you is to experiment with different strains, masturbate, and observe how they affect you. The next most reliable way is to go by the lab information that breaks down cannabinoid and terpene content, rather than relying on strain names or the now antiquated indica/sativa/hybrid designation. If stress and anxiety are getting in the way of pleasure and connection, try strains or products with a 1:1 ratio of THC to CBD. If you're trying to have high-energy, active sex, go with something that has a terpene profile that includes limonene (citrus aroma) or pinene (pine aroma). If you're looking for something slower and more sensual, pick a strain with linalool (floral aroma) or beta-caryophyllene (pepper aroma), which would likely be more relaxing."

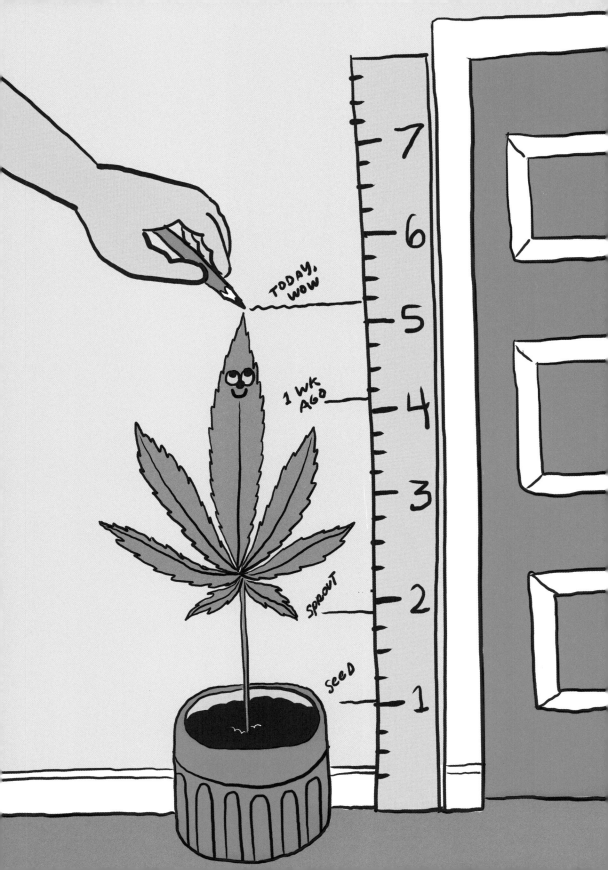

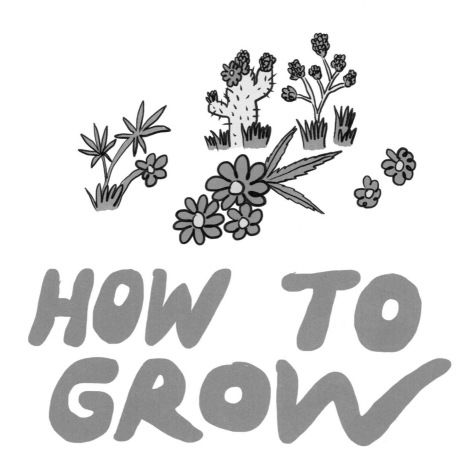

HOW TO GROW

Nothing tastes as good as a plant plucked from your own garden—or shoe closet. Growing your own weed is an eye-opening experience that deepens your relationship with it on a level that you could never achieve by simply walking into a dispensary and pointing your finger at a packaged product on a shelf.

As you feed and water your plants, you might even find yourself singing tenderly to your strains as you stroke their leaves, waiting for them to flower. Once they do, you'll be able to proudly smoke strains that you can guarantee are organic and pesticide-free.

You'll also have plenty of trim, shoots, and stems that you can use to make edibles, or even throw into a juicer to drink raw.

If you've ever looked at an empty corner of your basement or a spare plot in your garden and thought to yourself, "I could grow weed here," this chapter is for you. You should know that there are some risks involved—like electrical fires from hot lightbulbs, bug infestations, and moldy mildew. But I once met a pair of male model twins who shared a small room in Brooklyn and grew cannabis in their closet. If they can do it, you can too.

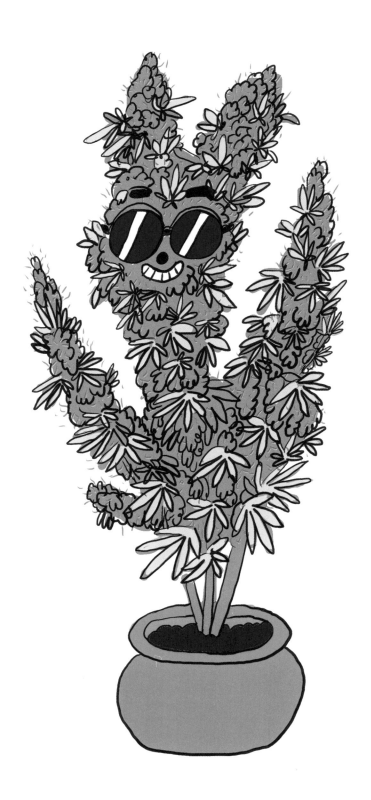

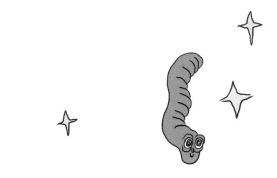

POT(TED) PLANTS: INDOOR GROWING

In nature, the cannabis plant only flowers once a year—usually when it becomes cold outside and the daylight hours get shorter. The part of the plant that we care about the most is the (female) flowers. To grow them, what you basically need to do is use an artificial light source to trick the plant into a growth cycle until it's mature and flowers, then harvest those juicy nugs—aka the dank buds of the flowers—so you can smoke them. These steps will give you a brief overview of how it works, but growing is a true craft that requires a lot of homework to succeed—I recommend *Grow Your Own* by Nichole Graf, Micah Sherman, David Stein, and Liz Crain as one of the best (and most fun-to-read) reference guides.

1. Set up your grow space

It should be somewhere cool, dry, and able to be sealed off completely from light. Whether a plant is male or female is genetically determined. Females will flower when they get twelve hours of light followed by twelve hours of darkness, but if light accidentally seeps into your grow room at the wrong time, the plants could return to a non-flowering state, or become intersex, due to stress. Set up your lights, keeping them low to the ground and adjusting them as the plant grows in height. Your plant is also going to need lots of CO_2, so make sure there's air circulating through the space, or set up fans in the corners.

2. Let the plant grow

This is the stage where the plant will sprout leaves and branches, but not flowers, yet. Ideally, a plant needs to grow for around four to six weeks before flowering or else it won't produce enough bud for your efforts to be really worth it. During this vegetative period, give your plant eighteen hours of light and six hours of complete darkness. Feed it lots of nutrients—or use a pre-fertilized soil mix—because good bud needs lots of nitrogen, phosphorus, and potassium. Be careful not to overwater, a common rookie mistake. To be safe, you can just wait until the leaves start to wilt a little before watering.

3. Harvest those nugs and hang them out to dry

Cut the branches off the plants and remove any unwanted leaves (saving them for other uses). Hang them up from a string or wire, or place them on a drying rack, in a dark room with temperatures of 60–70°F (15–21°C) and humidity between 44 and 55 percent (use a small fan to circulate the air). Leave them for five to fifteen days. The flowers are ready when they feel a little crisp on the outside and the smallest branches snap when you try to fold them.

GROW GEAR

The Basics:

Lights
250-watt HID (high-intensity discharge) bulbs—either HPS (high-pressure sodium) or MH (metal halide)—can be found in hardware stores for as little as $25. However, these bulbs do require a specialized HID fixture and/or ballast, as they don't screw into any standard home fixture safely. (These fixtures may run to as much as $200.) Note: 250 watts is on the weaker side, and you could go for higher-intensity lights if you want—but make sure you install and maintain them carefully so as not to start a fire.

Pot
Get a pot that will allow the soil to breathe, like a fabric pot or one with drainage holes, and a saucer. Remember to empty water run-off from the saucer regularly so the moisture doesn't attract bugs or mold.

Soil
Get an organic potting soil containing mild organic nutrients like guano or sea kelp (any material that will allow air to penetrate, like coco coir- or sphagnum-based mediums, are also excellent choices). Avoid salt-heavy synthetics like Miracle-Gro or other artificial nutrients. You're putting this in your body, after all.

If You Wanna Get Fancy:

Timer
To control when your lights go on and off (some might say this is actually an essential).

Fan
To help air circulate the space and reduce heat (those lights really do burn up).

Activated Carbon Filter
To eliminate odors (just in case you've got nosy neighbors).

Thermometer/Hygrometer
To keep track of temperature and humidity.

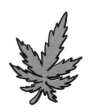

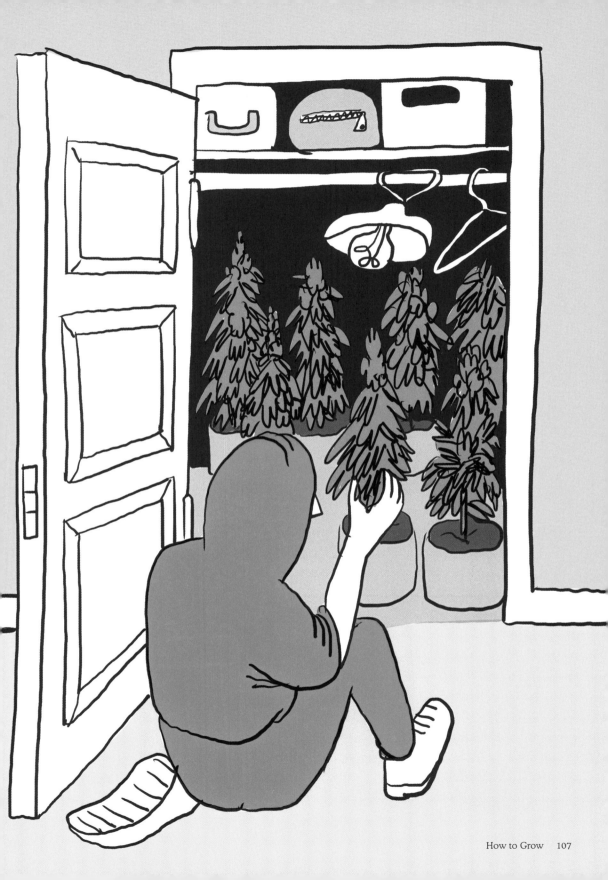

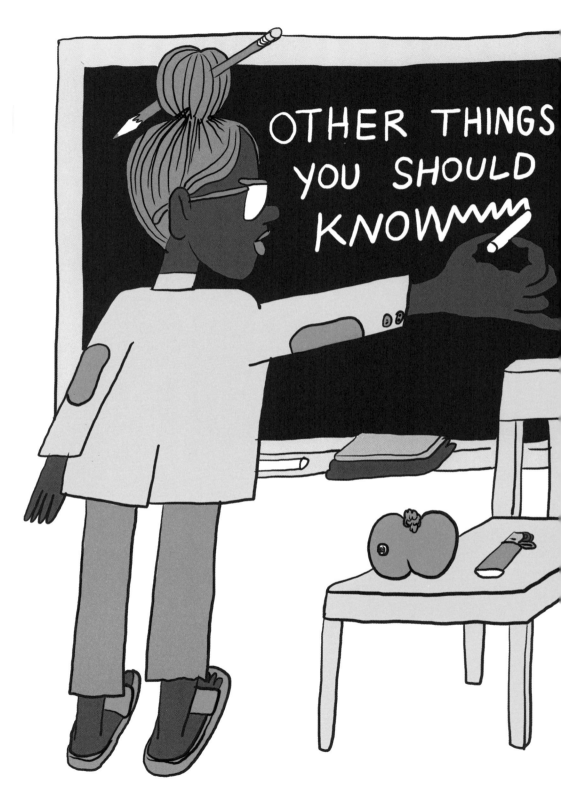

OTHER THINGS YOU SHOULD KNOW

Cannabis Seeds vs Clones

You can grow a weed plant using either cannabis seeds or clones—rooted cuttings that will be genetically identical to the plant they were taken from. Indoor growers tend to prefer clones because they're all female, so you don't have to cull out the males. Their "mother plants" have also been proven to produce good-quality bud, so you know exactly what effects and characteristics the strain will have. On the downside, the plants will be smaller and won't yield as much bud compared to growing from seed.

Curing

Storing your buds in an airtight container—a process called "curing"—after you've dried them out will help them stay potent for longer and smoke smoothly without that harsh, throat-burning feeling. During the first week, open the container a few times a day to let the flowers breathe. (If it smells weird, the bud isn't dry enough to be cured, so you should give it more time.) Two to three weeks of curing should suffice, but four to eight weeks is golden.

Growing Outdoors

Growing weed outdoors is not too different from indoors, except you have to water the plants more often (probably every day) and pay closer attention to any random hungry animals that might barge into your garden. (Indoor gardens, on the other hand, can be more susceptible to pests and mold.) Choose a spot that receives at least five to six hours of direct sunlight per day and is shielded from the wind. A month before you plant, dig a hole in the ground and fill it with compost from your kitchen, or with other decomposed organic matter. In addition to nutrients, this will help create the ideal soil composition to give the plant the proper aeration and water drainage that it needs.

Hydroponics

Hydroponics is an advanced, expensive, and very nerdy way to grow weed indoors that helps plants grow faster and with bigger yields of flowers. Basically, instead of nutrient-rich soil, you're feeding the roots concentrated solutions of mineral salt nutrients, using a setup involving air pumps and plastic tubing. The hydroponic process requires a lot of precision, because plants will be quicker to react to everything in their environment, including any mistakes you make —so this is definitely not for beginners.

CANNABIS FARMING WITH LISA LASER

At the end of every summer, when the weather gets crisper and the trees start to blush, thousands of migrant workers, or "trimmigrants," flock to weed farms for harvest season. In 2017, when a friend invited me to trim cannabis with him in the Emerald Triangle—a region in Northern California that grows more weed than anywhere else in America—I thought it sounded like a dream job. A journey into the center of the weed-growing world where you get to frolic in endless fields, smoke all day for free, *and* get paid thousands of dollars for a few weeks' work? It sounded too good to be true. "Nah," my friend said with a laugh. "Trimming *sucks*."

A few Google wormholes later, and I realized he was right. The internet is chock-full of warnings to wannabe trimmers who, like me, naively assume that working on a weed farm is a (stoned) walk in the park. First of all, you're stuck in the middle of nowhere for weeks, with no phone or internet service, living on very basic amenities, and doing tedious manual labor for twelve to sixteen hours every day. Even the steadiest diet of funny podcasts can't save you from the mind-numbing, back-breaking boredom. Second, many weed farms operate illegally on the edge of society, dodging authorities (as they have done for decades). A culture of paranoia wafts through the smoke as farm owners live in fear of getting raided or robbed.

Of course, this doesn't mean that all farms are dangerous—plenty are perfectly chill and run by good people. Still, I decided to hang back and wait for my friend to suss out the vibe so he could report back. A week or two later, he called: "It's over, everyone's been fired," he said glumly. Turns out the farm had decided to buy a bunch of trimming machines that were able to do the work for cheaper, so they let go of all the workers. I'd missed my chance.

I've always been curious about what I could have experienced, so I decided to hit up Lisa Laser, a highly respected grower. One of the few prominent women in the grow scene, Lisa runs a business selling cannabis clones from her nursery to other growers. Smoking a joint during one of her breaks, Lisa explained how to get a job on a weed farm, and shared some insider tips for growing cannabis yourself.

What brought you into the grow scene?
Coming from New York City, I knew that riding the subway every day with a briefcase was not going to make me happy. I went to college in Boulder, Colorado, and became a Grateful Dead hippie. I had a lot of friends who were growing pot—and this was back in 2007, when things weren't legal. I've always loved weed. My father passed away from cancer when I was thirteen, and when I started growing, I just felt as though I was doing

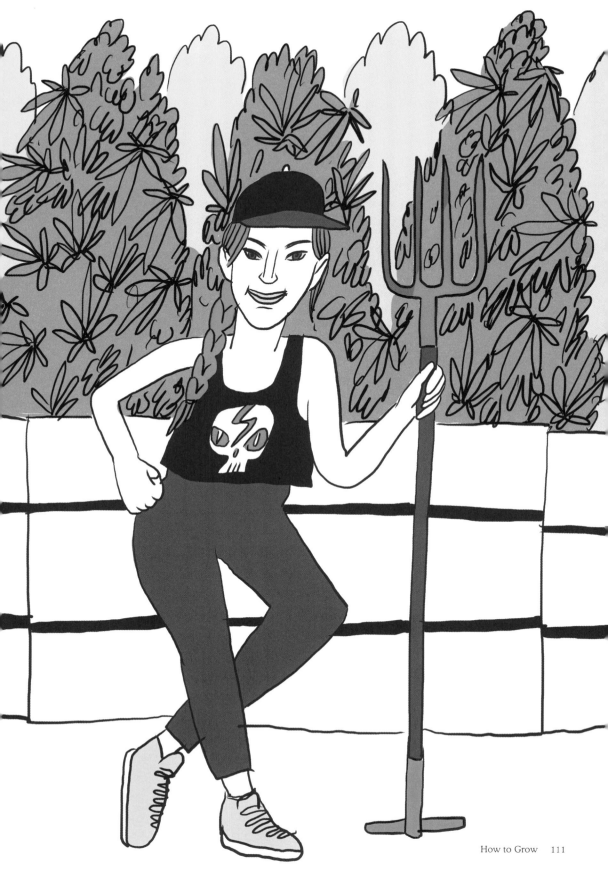

something right in terms of creating this medicine that I knew could help people. Later, my boyfriend and I decided to move to California and really take it to the next level as ganja growers. So I packed up and moved to the Santa Cruz Mountains with him.

You run a nursery selling clones. How do clones compare to seeds?
Clones are great for novice growers. They're pure replicas of each other, so every plant ends up exactly the same, which is great when you don't know what you're doing yet. A lot of full-sun outdoor growers like to start with seeds—but those can vary a lot in the aroma, the taste, and the way the plant grows.

Are you in the Emerald Triangle?
I'm actually in Grass Valley, which is between Sacramento and Tahoe. We have a really large grower community here as well. It's a little nook in Nevada County, California, that got overtaken by an influx of growers. In the Emerald Triangle there's not much to do other than grow—you're really in the sticks. Here, there's a cool community with music, food, outdoor activities, and a young community of people who get together. [The vibe is] pretty hippie-dippie, I'm not gonna lie. [There's] a lot of the Burning Man community, and artists. Then there's the conservative, agricultural community that was here before us.

Have there been any interesting trends in the grow world since legalization?
There's this new lean toward exotic-flavored weed. Farms need to provide variety like they never had to before, to be able to sell efficiently to the dispensaries. So instead of having two or three different strains, they're trying to have twenty-five, so that they can provide all these different, fun flavors to customers.

What kind of jobs are available to someone who wants to work on a weed farm?
There are different things that temp workers can do for hourly work. A lot of it begins with dirt work—getting new soil in and old soil out—that's something that [a newbie] could really get their

hands into. There's also always a ton of trim work. That's really what novice people can do, until they start to get the flow of being trusted with the plant. And then the harvest season is also a huge undertaking on large, commercial farms: getting everything down, hung up, and into the right environment quickly.

Is it easy to find work, or do you need to know people who can bring you into the scene?
There's been such an influx of growers into the ganja community in the last five years, and there's just every type of person in it. There are definitely some really shady people, and there are some wonderful people. That's why I think it's important to know the people you're working for are trustworthy. It's about using your common sense. My friends and I have [built] a rather large network of growers through the music community; I would never send someone somewhere if I didn't know exactly where they were going.

The other thing is that we have a lot of international trimmers coming into Northern California. Those people can get jobs by just hanging out at a local bar or coffee shop. You can kind of have a conversation and get work that way; but I think for the most part you have to know someone.

Are there any grow farms that are specifically for women?
I've found a few via Instagram, but they're few and far between. I think if the cutthroat-ness of the industry and the large egos that get attached to a lot of these grower guys [dipped], it would allow a lot more women to join in. Even though this industry is insanely male-dominated, I think if you're really focused and know your shit, you can get such a high level of support and respect. That's happening with me now, and it's opening my eyes to a different side of the industry. Now I have my own business and it's kind of flourishing, and everyone in my little town knows that I've been doing well.

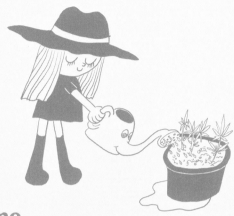

Lisa Laser's Tips for Growing Weed at Home

Read the grow bible
"I used to work at a grow store in Santa Cruz, and I had all these young college guys coming in asking me how to grow weed. The first thing I would always tell them is to read Jorge Cervantes's *Marijuana Horticulture: The Indoor/ Outdoor Medical Grower's Bible* cover to cover. It explains everything in understandable ways, and really goes through each step."

Poke around the internet
"You can really dork out and learn a lot just by reading and looking at photos, and from there, you can decide if you'd like to do a closet space or a garage space, for example."

Go to your local grow store
"Once you have an idea of what you want to do, go to your local grow store and ask the guys there to show you what they've got."

Less is more
"Not overwatering, overlighting, or overdoing anything is important. Remember, they're plants! A lot of newbies try almost too hard, adding too many nutrients or overwatering, which can cause root rot. Pruning plants too much is also something to be careful of."

Learn from your (and your friends') mistakes
"When you see something going wrong in your garden, take a solid look to see what's happening. When you hear about friends having problems, listen to what's going on so that you don't make those same mistakes."

Get on a simple watering schedule
"Nutrient companies give you week-by-week instructions for what, when, and how much you need to water. It's so helpful to go by those instructions, because their scientists have figured it out. I really like the House & Garden nutrient formula, but it's a bit expensive. For a cheaper one, I like the General Organics formula. Once you begin to get the hang of it, you can start tweaking and using different things."

Create the right environment in your room
"For any indoor grower, when you're first getting set up in a new space, dialing in your airflow and getting your temperature right with air conditioning and dehumidifiers can be a process. If you're trying to grow inside, you absolutely need to have your temperature controlled (see p. 105)."

Q&A

WHAT'S UP WITH WEED SCHOOL?

My friend Casey Jude and I went to the same high school when we lived in Singapore, a country notorious for its scarily strict drug laws. We both moved to America for college and continued living in the States. But during a trip back to Singapore a few months ago, I was leaving a techno club around 3 a.m. when I suddenly ran into Casey on the street. We ended up chilling on the sidewalk for a while, catching up, and he told me he was planning to go to the legendary Oaksterdam University, America's first cannabis college, founded in Oakland, California, in 2007. "Whoa, what's up with weed school?!" I wondered. So I decided to give Casey a call a few days after he graduated (on 4/20, the unofficial stoner holiday, obviously) to find out.

What made you decide to go to weed school?
I didn't like my job selling electronic manufacturing equipment for my dad, and was drinking too much. I realized I could transfer some of my skills [from my old job] to the cannabis industry, and the best way to ease myself into it was to go to Oaksterdam.

Why Oaksterdam specifically?
Oaksterdam was like an urban myth when I was going to the University of San Francisco, but I was too scared to go before weed was legal. When I signed up for Oaksterdam in late 2017, there were a couple of other weed craft schools, as well as four-year horticulture courses at universities. I figured a craft school would be best, and Oaksterdam is at the forefront of cannabis education.

A lot of our teachers are in the vanguard of the legal cannabis industry—they were at the protests, or filing the first business licenses for legal dispensaries in the Bay Area. With cannabis, you can get super-technical, but to learn about the industry through other people's experiences at Oaksterdam was pretty priceless.

At the same time, we're not creating new processes or learning about crazy, cutting-edge technology that's gonna change the industry. It's more about exploring the environment. We had field trips to cultivation sites, and meetings with practitioners, including guys who've been arrested for cannabis issues or have really hands-on experience.

How much does it cost and how do you get in?
I don't think they reject many people; admission's based on availability. They also help you with funding if you're not able to pay. I took two courses. The Classic course taught us the business aspects—licensing, legalities, lobbying, and the history of things like the Controlled Substances Act. That was $1,500. The Horticulture course was all hands-on with plants. You learned about nutrient sources, temperatures, late-flowering techniques, and how to make your own nutrients. That was $1,700. So my total for a semester—four months—was about $3,200.

Was it worth it?
I thought it was. Since the industry is expanding so fast, competition is crazy, so what's the best way to get hands-on experience? Work for somebody, or

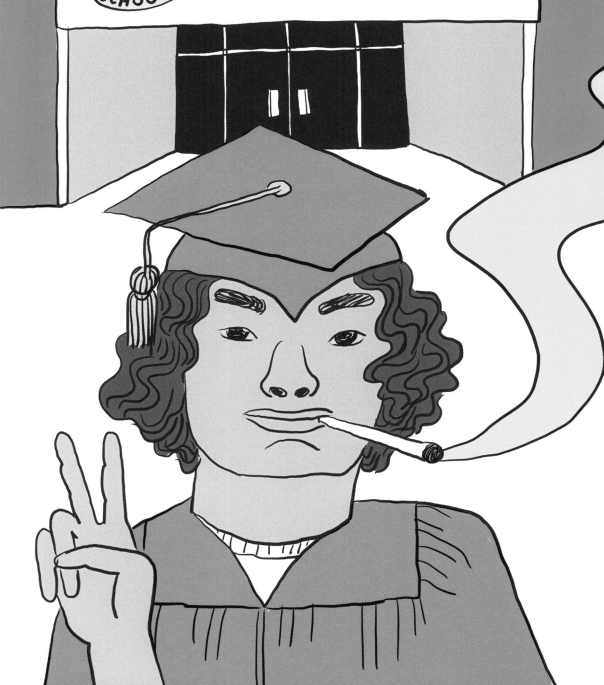

go to an educational institution and then pursue a job afterwards? I thought it was better to go to school because there are so many intricacies in the field right now. It's a weird time, and I wanted to know how I'd fit into the environment.

After going to Oaksterdam, I realized there are a lot of online certificates that are more narrow and focused, like a budtending certificate where you learn how to gauge someone's tolerance and not get them too high. But I think going to weed school will help me get a job. The Oaksterdam alumni network has forty thousand people in it. One of my friends got picked up right out of Oaksterdam and is now a manager at Hi-Fidelity [a cannabis dispensary in California]. He's hired a bunch of other Oaksterdam students.

Oaksterdam is also very social. We can talk about the technicalities, but the real thing about cannabis is the soft skills, and the sociability around it is really fun.

What were the other students like?
It was an eclectic mix. We had a far-right farmer from Sacramento; an ex-pro wrestler; a hobbyist from Germany who was rogue-growing; eighteen-year-olds straight out of high school; and this girl who moved to California to become a bud photographer. You really get everybody. There was even an older woman from the suburbs whose purpose was to learn how to lobby her own government—she and other seniors are growing pot for themselves, so they can provide other older people with safe access to marijuana.

How about the professors?
They get people to come in and teach what they do every day. A trademark lawyer came into the classroom to talk about trademarking $50,000 bongs. Outdoor growers taught us about the growth structures required to set up a greenhouse or outdoor grow operation. A woman who owns a CBD oil topical company talked about the medicinal and beauty value of CBD. Bakers talked about their journey selling baked goods on the black market and transitioning to a legal market.

One of the most legendary figures at Oaksterdam is Jeff Jones, who opened one of the first legal cannabis dispensaries in California. You could ask him anything you wanted about growing. We also had labs where we would learn how to trim and do other hands-on work with the plants—the campus has multiple grow tents.

Did anything surprise you?
It was a lot more work than I expected. I took two exams for each class, and the finals involved three hundred multiple choice questions. Throughout the course, you also have homework, and quizzes you have to take every day. On top of that, you have a final project of designing indoor and outdoor grow-ops. It'd be easy to go to weed school and get high all the time with your friends, but they really do help you learn and retain information. It's like any other college: what you put into it is what you get out.

What do you want to do next?
I've applied to jobs at companies like [cannabis farm collective] Madrone in California and [dispensary chain] MedMen (see p. 145) in New York. But my ultimate dream is to open a weed gallery where we'd throw art shows with paired weed strains—and a delivery service at night.

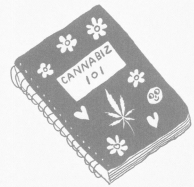

Where to Get a Higher Education

If you want to go to weed school:

Cannabis education centers
· Cannabis College
  (Amsterdam, the Netherlands)
· Clover Leaf University (Denver, Colorado)
· Humboldt Cannabis College
  (Humboldt County, California)
· Oaksterdam University (Oakland, California)
· Trichome Institute (Denver, Colorado)

If you want to take weed classes at
a "normie" school:

Universities with cannabis programs
· Harvard University
  (Cambridge, Massachusetts)
· Northern Michigan University
  (Marquette, Michigan)
· Ohio State University (Columbus, Ohio)
· University of Denver (Denver, Colorado)
· Vanderbilt University (Nashville, Tennessee)

If you don't want to leave your house:

Online-only programs
· 420 College (420college.org)
· Cannabis Career Institute
  (cannabiscareerinstitute.com)
· Cannabis Training University
  (cannabistraininguniversity.com)
· THC University (thcuniversity.org)
· TMCI Global
  (themedicalcannabisinstitute.org)

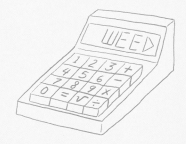

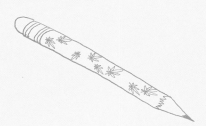

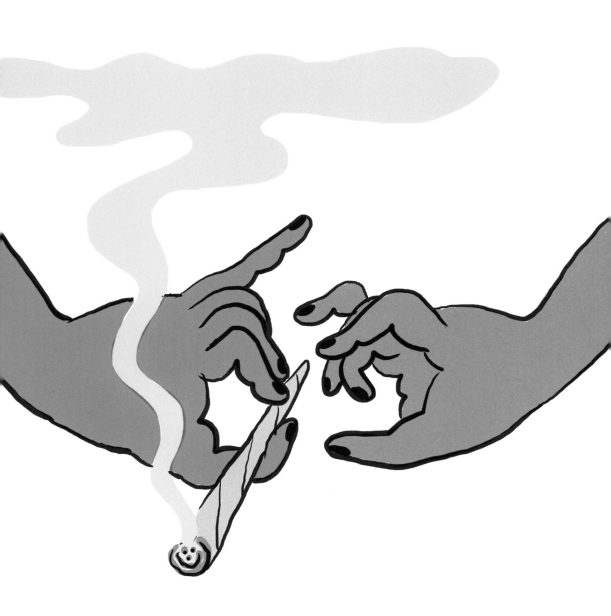

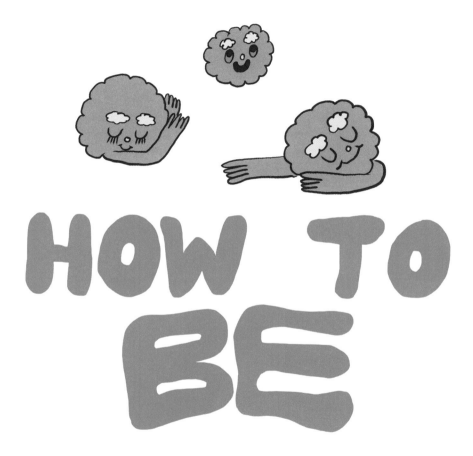

HOW TO BE

This is arguably the most crucial (and definitely my favorite) part of this book: how to be a proper stoner. Here, we'll go over etiquette and customs refined over generations of tokers—what you could consider "stoner code." These unspoken rules are grounded in a mix of common sense, hippie values, and basic respect, while also helping to prevent chaos or confusion in highly stoned situations. We'll go over the commandments of any smoke circle, cover the weird world of weed parties, and investigate the debate on how to inhale.

By the end of this chapter, you'll understand the correct protocol for passing a joint and how to join in a conversation on cannabis social issues while sounding woke AF. Because at the end of the day, weed is about more than knowing how to roll a nice blunt. It's a way of life, and this is how to do it right.

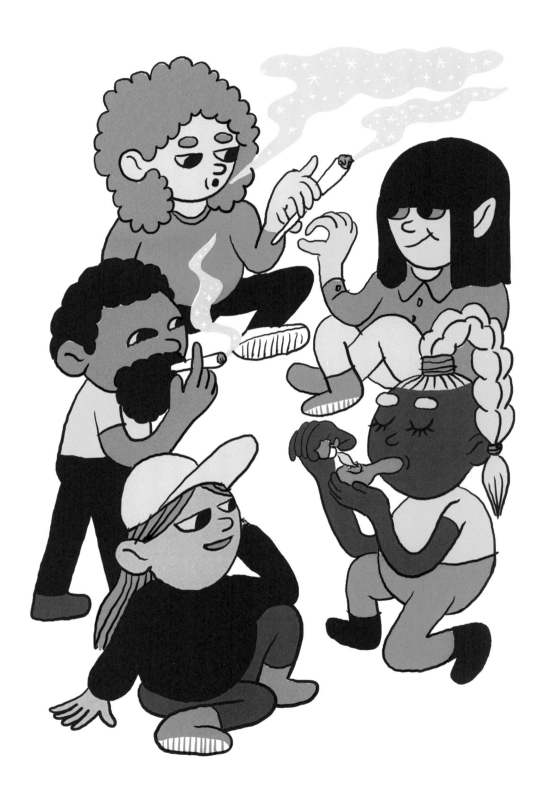

STONER CODE

What makes weed culture really special—and different from alcohol—is that it's based on hippie values like caring for each other. You never pressure someone to take a hit. You share pot freely without asking for payment or anything in return. More than perhaps any other drug, sharing is a huge part of stoner code. As long as you're respectful, you're allowed to ask strangers for a drag of their joint if you need it, like if you're at a rave and your stomach isn't feeling great.

By the same token, smoke people out by sharing weed whenever you can, and never accept money if someone offers it for a hit. Disclose if the weed is mixed with anything, including tobacco (in which case it's called a "spliff"). Graffiti kids are notorious for spiking their weed with angel dust (PCP), so if you're ever uncertain about what you're being offered, ask.

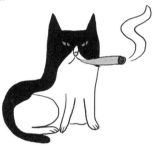

Smoke Circle Rules

1. The first hit is the greenest, so this treat should go to whoever supplied the weed or put in the most work—she who rolls it, sparks it. If you're sharing a bowl from a pipe, some extra-polite smokers even make sure to "corner hit" in order to leave some greens for the others.

2. Puff, puff, pass. Don't bogart the joint to tell a story while making everyone wait. Nobody cares—everyone's just thinking about smoking, so don't hold up the process. The general rule is "puff, puff, pass," but you can adjust this according to how many people are in your circle.

3. Always pass it to the left, moving in a clockwise direction. People sometimes break this one to pass it to their closest homie, but I'm a stickler for stoner code. Ash it before passing. Don't slobber on the joint, and smoke last if you're sick.

4. It's tacky to ask for the joint instead of waiting for your turn, but if someone's being really obnoxious, try a more subtle route by nodding toward the joint and asking, "Hey … is that lit?" They should get the hint.

5. Never waste weed! Don't put out the joint before checking if anyone wants the last hit, and if you're really hardcore, save your roaches. You can dump them out later to make a perfectly good and very economical joint—trust me, you'll thank me the next time you're out of weed.

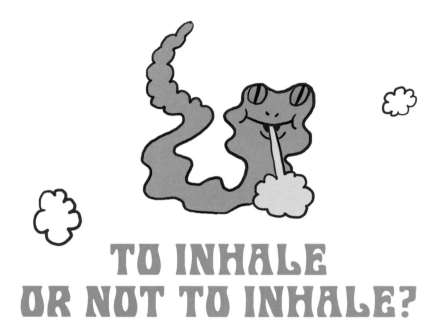

TO INHALE OR NOT TO INHALE?

For generations, you weren't considered a real stoner unless you knew how to inhale by holding the smoke deep in your lungs for a few seconds. Coughing was almost considered part of the ritual of proper smoking. Bill Clinton infamously said he smoked when he was young but didn't inhale (lame). Barack Obama, on the other hand, admitted he inhaled … because that's the point.

However, new research suggests that full THC absorption occurs within milliseconds, which means that holding smoke in your lungs for a prolonged period only results in absorbing more carcinogens from weed smoke (unless you're vaping). So maybe just holding smoke in your mouth can get you as stoned, and inhaling actually does the opposite of what you're intending to do: waste weed. Still, most potheads today will give you skeptical looks if you blow out too quickly.

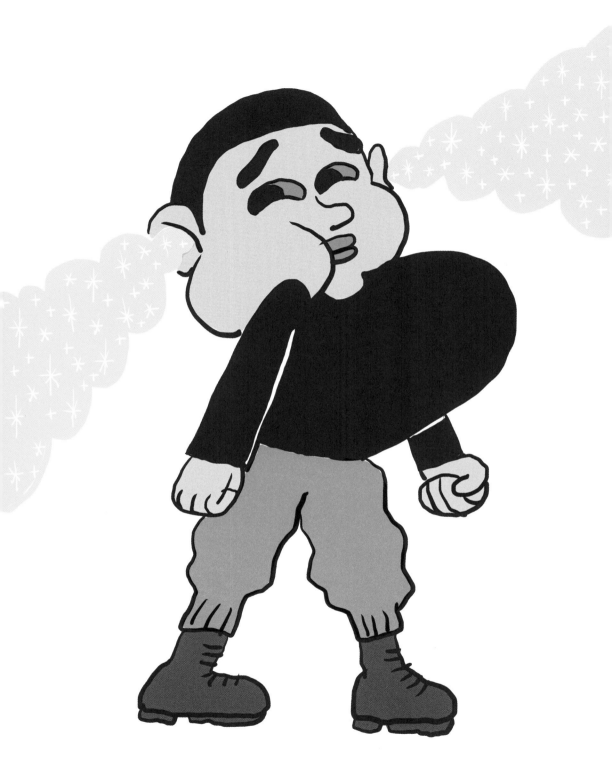

INTERVIEW WITH ANJA CHARBONNEAU AND STEPHANIE MADEWELL OF BROCCOLI MAGAZINE

I've been digging the feminist weed magazine *Broccoli* ever since the cover of their first issue went viral in late 2017. The striking image showed an example of the traditional Japanese floral arrangement method *ikebana*, but instead of flowers, the magazine's florist had used long stalks of stems and leaves from a cannabis plant. For the first time, I saw the weed leaf in a new light—and was struck by how elegant it could be. I became so obsessed that I set the photo as my phone's screensaver.

"The pot leaf feels like a tired symbol because you associate it with the T-shirt at the corner street market," says *Broccoli* founder Anja Charbonneau over the phone from Portland. "The coolest thing about reinterpreting something so well known is to show people there's another way of looking at things."

Beyond defining a new kind of weed aesthetic, though, that cover image also represents *Broccoli*'s new way of talking and thinking about weed. Editor-in-chief Stephanie Madewell and her team love to highlight women whose contributions to cannabis culture often go under-recognized, and offer articles that span beyond typical pothead fare. When it comes to stoner culture, Charbonneau says, "You thought you knew what this was—but there's actually a much bigger story unfolding."

What are some of the most interesting trends you've noticed in the weed industry?
AC: I'm really excited about all the upcoming medical and scientific research initiatives now

that there's more room to study weed. There's a [tendency] to say more than we actually know scientifically about cannabis. People love to say you can take this product for this result, but we're really not there yet. Every time there's new information, everyone jumps on it, because it's one more piece to this puzzle that we're all slowly working together to solve. We want to go beyond the anecdotes. On a science and consumer level, people want that knowledge. And it's coming soon, hopefully.

SM: One of the fascinating things about cannabis is you have so many people using it for so many different reasons. The attorney leading the case to get marijuana's Schedule I drug classification [in the US] changed recently quoted a statistic that 96 to 98 percent of Americans are in favor of some form of legalization. We can't agree on anything in this country, and it's wild that we can agree on this. Conservative people are on the same side as coastal liberal elites. This agreement is something people are waking up to.

Are there interesting cultural variations in attitudes, or ritualistic ways that people consume weed, across different countries or state lines?
AC: One of the most exciting things when we launched the magazine was that we started to hear stories from women all over the world—in Hong Kong, South Africa, Latvia ... For a lot of them, it was their first opportunity to connect with women with whom they had this thing in common, because maybe where they live it's not super-common. These women really want legal

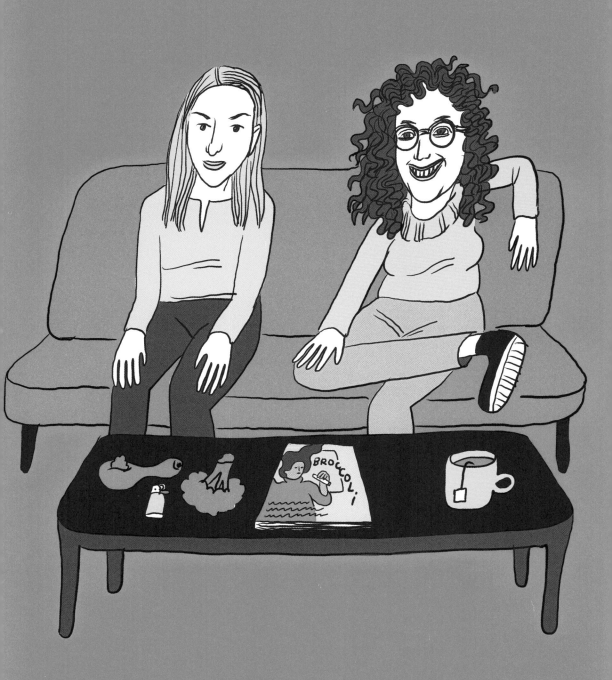

weed, they want to have the knowledge that their cannabis is being grown safely and ethically and organically, and they're not supporting a narco-drug trade. We have a lot of readers in Brazil who struggle with this. Unless you're growing it yourself or have a network of growers, it's hard to get a safe, quality product. I see that as something people are wanting across the world. They look at the legal states in the US with some admiration and hope. We have so much responsibility to set a good example, because people from all over the world are watching us to see how it's done. And if we can set good examples, there'll be a really nice domino effect throughout the world as more countries start to legalize.

Do you think women approach weed differently from men?
AC: Women are coming together more as a community to talk about their experiences and how cannabis fits into their lives. That feels very unique. Sharing personal experiences is something women tend to be more versed in. In cannabis, where anecdotal experiences are all we have right now, that's infinitely valuable.

SM: Women are served terribly by the medical community; there's a huge, unmet need for care for women's health issues. Women in cannabis are creating businesses and sharing stories to help each other out, saying, "If you suffer from this, this is what has helped me."

Why do you think the cannabis industry has been so welcoming to female entrepreneurs?
AC: I'm on the other side of this issue—I find the numbers to be really bad, and not something we should be proud of. There was a popular study in *Marijuana Business Daily* in 2015 that said that women make up 36 percent of leadership roles within the cannabis space, while the national industry average is 21 percent. There was a wave of positivity surrounding that number. What people haven't noticed is that the same group updated that number last year, and there was a drop of 9 percent, down to 27 percent. A survey is never going to be the be-all, end-all picture of the industry. I'm really interested in seeing how many women actually own businesses in the cannabis industry, because that's where you'll see real change coming from. When you track things back to the owners, you'll usually find that it's a man making all the decisions.

There's a lot of amazing work being done by women, and they're having their voices heard more than we're used to. But on the other hand, cannabis is falling into outdated and unjust patterns. I worry that there are more structural injustices coming into cannabis from corporate industries than we're really noticing.

SM: It's also really telling that people are so happy about the 36 percent, because it's kind of crappy given that we're half the population. We deserve to not be happy with the crumbs of success.

What can we do to make things better?
AC: There's so much room to celebrate what women are doing in cannabis, but we have to follow up that celebration with a lot of action. That could look like going into a dispensary and asking the budtender which products come from women-owned farms or businesses. This encourages people who are making decisions on any level of a cannabis company to think about equality. If you start asking for it, people will listen, because they want to be ethical businesses.

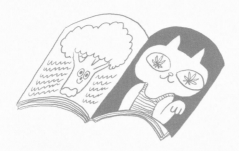

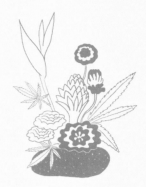

Broccoli's Tips on How to Start Your Own Weed Platform

Establish a clear set of values
"This makes business and editorial decisions easier because you have a sense of what you want to do, and the voice you want to be in the world. First, question if you want to create your own platform: why do you want to do that? Having that sense of intention is not something you can buy or make up—it's either there for you or it's not, and it's really important. With the cannabis industry expanding, you have a market of ideas and values."

Know what audience you want to reach
"Cannabis is becoming more targeted, so knowing who you're talking to and what stories you want to tell is the first step. You have to do a lot of listening and paying attention, and really understand your audience and where they're at, what they're into."

Bring your own sensibility to it
"Without pandering, you want to take others' interest and passion as a starting place, and pull in your own influences and inspiration. Bringing a fresh perspective and sense of discovery to your subjects: that's what'll make it unique and compelling."

Work hard to secure diverse voices
"Don't bother starting a media platform if you're only hiring people that are like you. Unless you're working with writers from different countries and backgrounds, you're not gonna be telling stories that are relevant to the rest of the world."

Get money
"While it might look like cannabis is a gold rush, it's really hard for companies to find their footing as legalization unfolds. In Oregon, where I [Anja] live, we've been recreationally legal for a couple of years, but there are still little rule changes that affect companies in big ways.

Not everyone has the resources to fund their own projects. You have to decide if you want to sell to readers with a subscription fee, or work in partnerships, or work with an investor. None of these are easy. On a brand level, we're looking for funders who share the same ethos and want to support the same vision: those interested in quality and honesty, with an eye for design. Look for someone who believes in what you're doing, and whose background you really respect—if you're giving up part of the ownership of your company, you want to go into that with someone who has good intentions. They'll have a voice now, so you have to be careful."

Watch the response you get from the world
"We're seeing a community unfold for us that we didn't expect. We need to have the ability to listen and adapt, and be responsive to that opportunity."

THE PEOPLE YOU'LL MEET AT A WEED PARTY

A strange new phenomenon has been popping up all over the world: weed parties. These events, usually thrown by cannabis companies, can take all forms: wild mansion bacchanals, meditative sound baths, lavish dinners, dance parties with DJs ... Really, the only thing they have in common is lots of free dank bud. And if you follow your favorite weed brands on social media, you're bound to get invited to one soon enough.

Once you're in, you'll be thrust into a strange milieu of stoner stereotypes from every corner of the weed world. You'll start to notice that certain types of people are always at these things, smoking joints by the pool, swarming the tables of freebies, picking at the empty buffet. Each creature in this eccentric kingdom has their own distinct characteristics, and before you approach, you should know how to identify them—and what to watch out for.

So here's a handy reference guide to the six types of stoners you'll meet at a weed party.

1. The Creepy Industry Dinosaur

The Creepy Industry Dinosaur has been in the "cannabiz" since before it got all mainstream—and they will make sure you know that, by saying stupid things like "cannabiz." They all know each other from Cannabis Cup '88 and will incessantly tell you how much crazier things were back in those wild days, while offering you their (admittedly very dank and plentiful) stash of weed as a way to try and sleep with you. Fortunately, these types always know everyone over forty at the party and get distracted, so it's easy to escape their clutches and slip away.

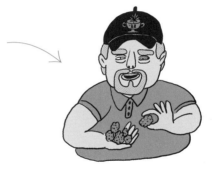

2. The Overeager Publicist

Weed publicists didn't really exist a decade ago, if you think about it—there were essentially no legal products to push. But good timing and connections have landed these people in one of the buzziest, fastest-growing (and most competitive) industries in the world—and they are stoked!!! You'll usually find the Overeager Publicist at the door, cheerfully welcoming celebrity guests while keeping an eye out for gatecrashers. Don't let their wide smiles fool you. They're the gatekeepers to this scene, and boy, do they know it. Still, it's always a good idea to play nice and smile back, since you want to be invited to the next party—and they usually have a bunch of extra freebies to throw your way.

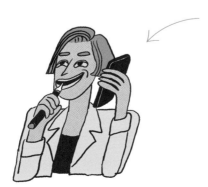

3. The Bored Party Girl

The Bored Party Girl—who can also take the form of a fabulous gay boy—is here to get good #content for their Instagram Stories and get really, really baked before they head off to the next rave. They can be seen aimlessly wandering around in pairs, clutching each other's elbows while whispering, "Where's the free weed?!" "I don't know, but why is there no one *hot* here?!" As they weave through the crowd in search of weed swag, their tattoos, skin-tight mesh tops, and plastic platforms glimmer through the clouds of bong smoke. After a few hours of freeloading, they get bored and leave.

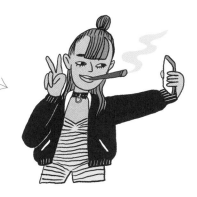

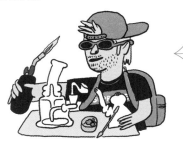

4. The Nerdy Dab Bro

The Nerdy Dab Bros only came to this party because they wanted to check out the latest pneumatic dual-heat rosin press machine that they have been debating over in the /r/dailydabbers subreddit. They consider themselves cannabis concentrate connoisseurs, own at least three electronic dabbers, and laugh at anyone still smoking out of old-fashioned pipes, which they snidely call "analogs." Backpack, backwards cap, and T-shirt with some lame weed pun like "Just Hit It" are their aesthetic. Probably owns a membership to Hitman Coffee Shop (see p. 146).

5. The Hip-Hop Mogul

Rolls up in a Rolls-Royce smoking two blunts and is immediately escorted by the Overeager Publicist, who is practically bowing down at their feet, to the VIP section by the pool, which gets closed off to everyone except the Mogul's entourage of CEO friends for an impromptu photo shoot. Their presence sucks the air out of the room as everyone stops what they're doing to turn around and low-key gawk at their shenanigans. Usually found draped in Louis Vuitton scarves, thousand-carat jewelry, and glassy-eyed models, smoking strains grown by their homie "Wiz" (Khalifa).

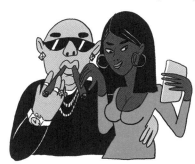

6. The Earthy Bohemian

These non-GMO, organic, and sustainable raw vegans are here because their third eye told them to be. "May the light in me shine on the light in you," they tell you—stealing the phrase from their last yoga instructor—as they pass a joint rolled with lavender and kratom with a warm smile. These types think of weed as a "sacred ritual," say "elevated" instead of "stoned," and will try to get you to come to their next "elevated art experience" event with reiki healing and CBD massages (which somehow cost a bunch).

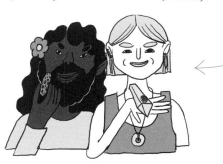

Q&A

TAO LIN ON WRITING ABOUT CANNABIS

Artists are prone to imbibing all kinds of drugs to summon the fickle winds of inspiration, but weed might be their favorite muse. Cannabis and creativity go hand in hand: it can help you feel more open, vulnerable, and experimental, or even help you make associations you might not have otherwise. From Shakespeare to the Beat poets, many of the greatest writers of every generation have taken a few puffs before facing themselves on the page.

Tao Lin is a New York-based writer whom many look up to as an icon in the "alt-lit" scene—a loose community of young writers who draw from internet culture in their work. In 2018 he published his first non-fiction book, *Trip: Psychedelics, Alienation, and Change*, which chronicles his journey as he turns away from pharmaceutical drugs like Xanax and Adderall—which he'd long used to soothe his anxiety and depression—and toward cannabis and psychedelic drugs like LSD and DMT.

Lin's plunge into weed and psychedelics began when he discovered the work of Terence McKenna, an American author and mystic-like figure in the 1980s and '90s experimental drug scene who spent his life championing the power of psychedelic plants. *Trip* begins with Lin taking a plant-drawing class under McKenna's former partner Kathleen Harrison, before delving into

how his own self-experimentation with plants transformed him from living in an opiate-fueled, "zombie-like" state to viewing the world with a sense of wonder.

In the midst of a tour of cities across America to promote his new book, Lin shared his insights into the relationship between weed and creativity.

How does weed affect your thought process and emotions when you're trying to be creative?
It gives me another state of consciousness for creating writing or drawings. I feel more emotional and am more moved by love and interactions; the experience of writing and drawing can be more enjoyable, intense, and compassionate while stoned. If I'm completely sober, I don't enjoy writing or drawing, so it's harder to do it.

In *Trip*, you write that weed helps you see the world with "unselfconscious, appreciative eyes." How does this sense of awe affect the way you process the world and put it into writing?
I think it actually takes me away from writing. It makes me write less, because seeing my computer screen with "unselfconscious, appreciative eyes" doesn't really help me at all. It helps me when I'm trying to interact with friends or nature—to focus on enjoying them, instead of worrying, feeling self-conscious, and mired in my own thoughts.

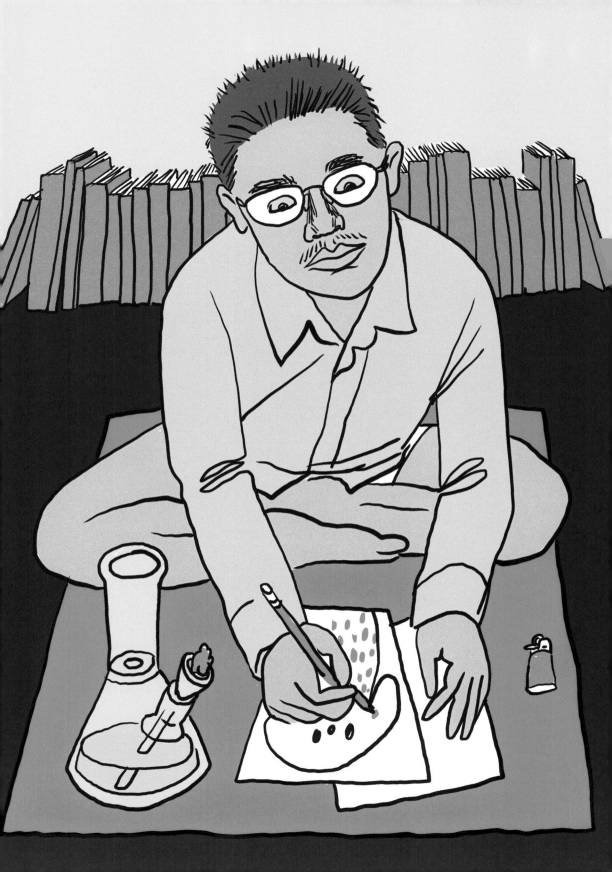

What are some of the funniest, weirdest, most random things you've written or created stoned?

Since I've been stoned every day—except sometimes while in Taiwan, or for isolated days in other countries—since September 2013, I would say the funniest thing I've created while stoned might, to me, be *Trip*'s DMT chapter, in which I become very paranoid for two or three hours and think my friend is a CIA agent or journalist trying to frame me.

What is your preferred ritual for consuming weed when you want to be creative and productive?

This is hard to answer, because I want to be creative and productive all the time, every day—and I have been. Writing *Trip*, I worked every day for an average of eight hours. So my ritual was just to wake up, drink coffee, smoke weed, and start working. But in 2017, I started smoking around five hours after waking, so now I can work on caffeine, not stoned, then work stoned later.

A water bong has worked best for me. Vaporizers have worked worst, even though I still like them— worst because they seem to break easily, and often I feel like I'm not getting stoned enough, fast enough. I have sometimes prayed to cannabis by just closing my eyes and thanking it, but it hasn't become ritualized. I've only done this maybe five times.

Do you think weed is helpful for common writers' ailments like writer's block, creative anxiety, and burnout? Are there scenarios where it might hinder your ability to write (for example, weed hangovers or bad time management)?

If I haven't smoked in two hours, smoking will get me motivated again. [But] I've been hindered by weed when I've gotten too stoned. This happened somewhat often while writing *Trip*. At some point, I'd start getting too stoned to work on writing or even to edit, at which point I would draw. Maybe only once or twice, when I've had edibles and smoked, have I been too stoned to draw. But I was able to control that and stop it.

Do you think you're most creative when you get stoned with a vape, edible, joint, or dab?

I'm most creative when I've had a lot of sleep and sunlight and then use weed—for writing, probably a vape, joint or edible. Writing—typing words in a row—is so linear and somewhat constricted, so I feel I can get too stoned using dabs or wax or a strong edible for it to be ideal for writing.

There's a famous Hemingway quote: "Write drunk, edit sober." Is there a difference in the way you approach writing versus editing with weed?

I write and edit both stoned and not stoned, and on caffeine and tobacco, and other drugs. My quote would be: "Write sober and stoned, edit sober and stoned." Also, write and edit in other states of consciousness, so you can keep seeing your work differently, and keep working on it.

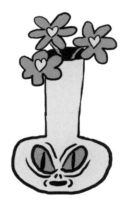

Tao Lin's Favorite Weed Books

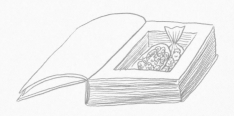

Cannabis and Spirituality: An Explorer's Guide to an Ancient Plant Spirit Ally, anthology edited by Stephen Gray, 2017

"This collection of essays by eighteen modern cannabis users explores how the plant can be used for spiritual purposes. It is worth reading in particular for Kathleen Harrison's contribution, 'Who Is She?,' which examines the use of cannabis to enhance gratitude or creativity. 'Muses tend to hug the edges, and are invoked via quiet rituals and personal patterns of invocation,' she writes, 'That is one of the gifts that cannabis offers—to be a muse for those of us who wish to contemplate and understand, or perhaps spend a little time just appreciating the mystery of it all.'"

PiHKAL: A Chemical Love Story by Alexander Shulgin and Ann Shulgin, 1991

"*PiHKAL* by Alexander and Ann Shulgin, the godparents of the modern psychedelic scene, is over seven hundred pages long and includes profiles, trip reports, and histories of DMT, LSD, DiPT, and other psychedelics. The Shulgins didn't enjoy cannabis, even though they loved a wide range of psychedelics—they say it has a 'stoning' effect that isn't productive for them. 'A stoning effect … is characterized, usually, by a general inability and disinclination to deal with concepts or to employ insight. In other words, one finds it difficult to learn anything of value,' they write in *PiHKAL*'s glossary. It is interesting to get a different perspective on cannabis from the Shulgins—one opposite to my own experience."

True Hallucinations: Being an Account of the Author's Extraordinary Adventures in the Devil's Paradise by Terence McKenna, 1993

"Terence McKenna called himself the most assiduous smoker of cannabis that he'd ever met.

He smoked—hash and cannabis—morning to night, almost every day, for more than twenty-five years. He stopped once, for months, and said it didn't affect him at all. But when I talked to [his ex-wife] Kathleen Harrison in 2016, she said that when Terence went off cannabis, he was nightmarish to be around—no sense of humor, grumpy, and so on. *True Hallucinations* is arguably McKenna's masterpiece. In it, he writes about traveling to the Amazon with his brother and some friends to search for a DMT-containing drug used by the Witoto people. Instead, they found psilocybin mushrooms, which they later learned how to grow, publishing their technique in *Psilocybin: Magic Mushroom Grower's Guide* in 1976."

Sisters of the Extreme: Women Writing on the Drug Experience, anthology edited by Cynthia Palmer and Michael Horowitz, 2000

"Women are often left out of drug culture, and published accounts of their views on cannabis and other psychedelics seem somewhat rare. This anthology of women writing about their drug experiences, including Maya Angelou on cannabis and Kathleen Harrison on salvia, helps to correct the imbalance. Published in 2000, it includes a history of cannabis as well as one on psychedelics by the editors, and is the expanded, second edition of 1982's *Shaman Woman, Mainline Lady*."

A Really Good Day: How Microdosing Made a Mega Difference in My Mood, My Marriage, and My Life by Ayelet Waldman, 2017

"Waldman's book is focused on microdosing LSD for one month, after every other type of medication she tried failed to combat her severe mood swings. But Waldman also writes about cannabis as part of her experiment, and how she began using it, instead of pills, to help her sleep."

LEE "SCRATCH" PERRY ON POT AND MUSIC

Over the last fifty years, Lee "Scratch" Perry, the eighty-two-year-old "godfather of dub," has been called a lot of things: mad scientist, reggae shaman, cultural icon, and "the Salvador Dalí of music," as The Rolling Stones' Keith Richards put it. In the early 1970s, Perry built a DIY studio in his backyard in Kingston, Jamaica, that he called the "Black Ark." Everyone from Bob Marley and the Wailers to Junior Marvin came to jam in that studio, and the techniques he used back then still blow people's minds.

Perry—with his bright-red goatee, jewel-encrusted robes, and assortment of elaborate hats that puts the Kentucky Derby to shame—is a cross between genius music producer and mystic. His wildly experimental techniques often have a whiff of the occult: he would blow weed smoke over tapes, bury microphones under palm trees to create drum effects, and record samples using the kitchen utensils, broken bottles, and barbed wire he'd decorate his mixing boards with.

Along the way, Perry pioneered a multilayered, reverb-drenched style of dub music—a bass-heavy offshoot of reggae—that he compared to "the ghost in me coming out." Everyone from the Beastie Boys to Kanye West has been influenced by Perry. Without the production techniques he invented, which involved a lot of distortion, echoes, and backward tape looping, there's a good chance hip-hop, reggae, and rock wouldn't sound the way they do.

Perry burned down the Black Ark in 1978 but has never ceased his sonic explorations. He won a Grammy in 2003, and went on tour last year with Subatomic Sound System to celebrate the re-release of his 1976 album *Super Ape*—a stoner classic whose cover featured a giant gorilla holding a fat joint.

When I called Perry one afternoon in 2014 for an interview for *VICE*'s music website, he was living back in Jamaica, and his husky, Patois-laced voice

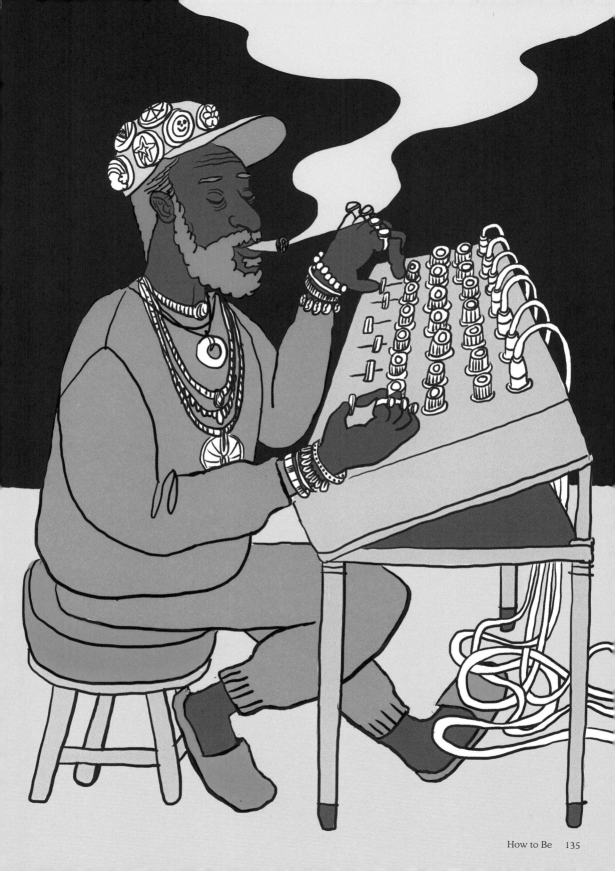

crackled through the phone line. His answers to my questions were more like cryptic riddles full of mystical references and wordplay; many of his sentences rhymed. He sang me the Happy Birthday song (it wasn't my birthday), and even led me in a prayer to bless our poop.

He also told me back then that he'd quit smoking weed. "I discovered my lungs are crying out for help," he said. "So I stopped smoking and started exercise. Sexercise. In bed. I started sexercising in bed, and more exercising in my head." But recently, I read online that he'd started getting stoned again, and wondered what had changed. So I hit up Perry for another illuminating interview—and his responses, once again, are a madcap delight.

Why do you think reggae music and ganja go together so well?
Because they are the same spirit. Ganja and one Jah. One aim, one flame, and one destiny.

When you blow ganja smoke over your tapes, what kind of effect does it have?
It's a genie. The smoke is a genie and the ganja is a genie and the electricity is a genie. So they work together to make magic.

Why did you decide to start smoking ganja again?
Because too much of one thing is good for nothing. If you do too much of one thing, you have to make a change and start all over again. When you overdo things, you have to start all over again to find a middle.

What do you think about the legalization of weed happening all over America and the rest of the world?
It goes to prove that ganja is a fateful doctor. Nothing is impossible to ganja. Ganja can make everything that is impossible, possible. Ganja is a genie and a god and a king. Ganja is a prince. Ganja is a king. Ganja is the Emperor Rastafari. But the business of ganja has a problem. The ganja needs a company so that it has the sun, the moon, the clouds, and the sky to back it. The government legalize ganja only to make money, tax money.

What's your favorite ganja recipe?
Ganja is good for fever and to conquer virus. Ganja, cerasee [bitter melon] tea, and ginger. Cook it in boiling water for half an hour. After, strain it and put the liquid in a bottle with lime juice. Also, mix ganja with white rum and lime, and drink it. It is a cure, a medicine.

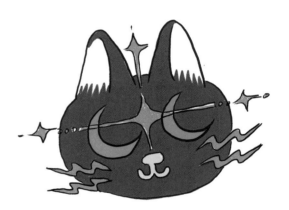

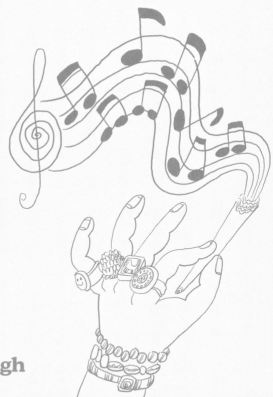

What to Listen to High

Iconic songs written by stoners, for stoners.

Reggae
"Kaya" by Bob Marley
"Legalize It" by Peter Tosh
"Sinsemilla" by Black Uhuru

Metal
"Dopesmoker" by Sleep
"Rosetta Stoned" by Tool
"Sweet Leaf" by Black Sabbath

Electronic
"Dutch Flowerz" by Skream
"Marijuana" by DJ Sneak
"Rollup" by Flosstradamus

Jazz
"Let's Go Get Stoned" by Ray Charles
"Pot Hound Blues" by Lucille Bogan
"The Reefer Man" by Cab Calloway

Classic Rock
"Light My Fire" by The Doors
"Panama Red" by New Riders of the Purple Sage
"Purple Haze" by The Jimi Hendrix Experience

'90s Rock
"Hash Pipe" by Weezer
"Moist Vagina" by Nirvana
"Smoke Two Joints" by Sublime

Country
"High Time" by Kacey Musgraves
"It's All Going to Pot" by Willie Nelson
    and Merle Haggard
"Roll Another Number (For the Road)"
    by Neil Young

Hip-Hop
"I Wanna Get High" by Cypress Hill
"The Next Episode" by Dr. Dre
    (featuring Snoop Dogg)
"Pass That Dutch" by Missy Elliott

Pop
"2 On" by Tinashe
"Dooo It!" by Miley Cyrus
"James Joint" by Rihanna

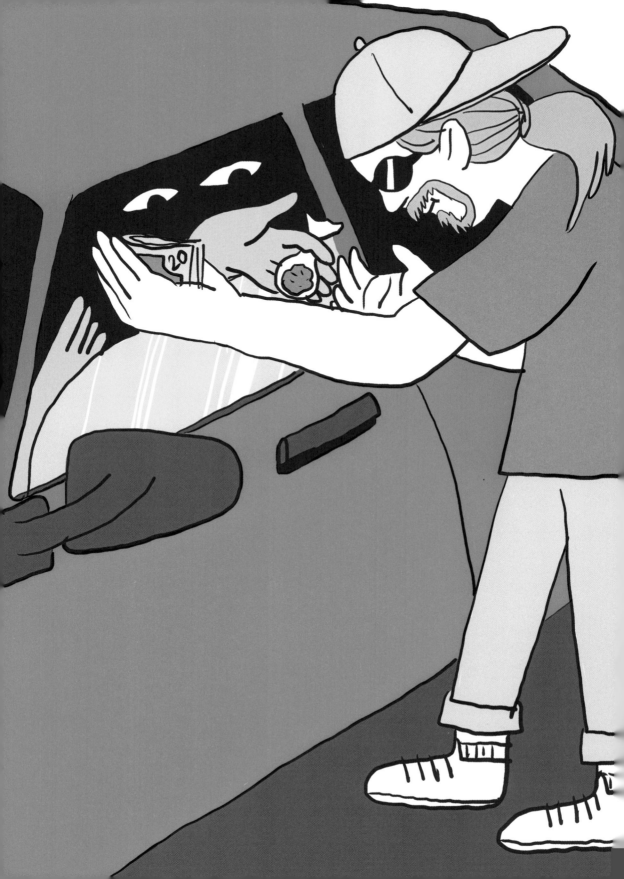

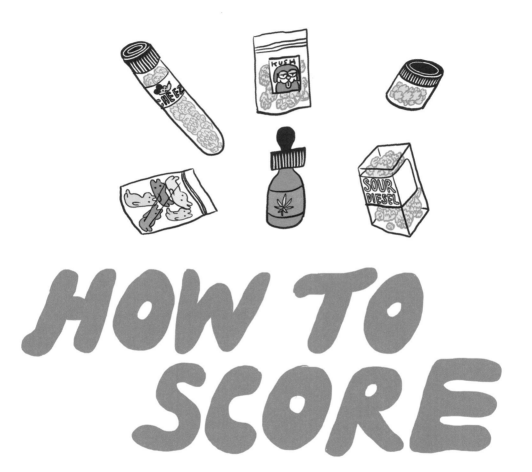

HOW TO SCORE

Everything we've talked about in this book is basically useless if you don't know where to get weed. While you could probably find a friend's-friend's-friend willing to sell you a stash within three text messages, we're going to focus on both brick-and-mortar businesses and online stores. We'll start with some of the most unique (medical and recreational) dispensaries in the world—weed stores that double as celebrity art galleries, DIY museums, or even have drive-throughs for your car. Then we'll jump into the best cannabis cafés and private lounges—social spaces that let you hang out with fellow stoners and stuff your face with food. Finally, we'll go over the best websites for cool accessories, home delivery, and even strain reviews. In this brave new age of weed, with so many resources at your fingertips, you have little excuse for finding yourself stuck in a sketchy car on the side of the street buying shake.

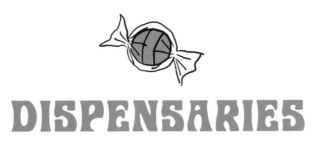

DISPENSARIES

The first dispensary I ever went to was in Los Angeles in 2015, pre-legalization. I was on a shoot for *VICE*'s show *Munchies* and was asked to get a medical card, which turned out to be just a piece of paper with a cheap golden seal, from a bro-like doctor who seemed very stoned. With my new card I was able to hit up any dispensary, but what struck me is how sketchy it still felt—metal doors, intimidating bouncers, no exterior signage.

Some dispensaries are still kind of weird, and most remain cash-only, but many shiny new businesses are like Willy Wonka Chocolate Factories for adults—full of unfathomable delights and unexpected discoveries.

The Silicon Valley Hub
What: Elemental Wellness Center
Where: San Jose, California

What's the deal: There's nowhere on earth quite like Elemental, a cannabis center with a vibe somewhere between a fancy gym and Silicon Valley coworking space—purple walls, shelves of merch, lots of computers. You can get a free massage, yoga class, or acupuncture here. That's pretty much all you need to know.

What to get: Elemental is famously the home of True OG—an extremely dank, award-winning indica that's one of the most potent strains out there (Elemental's nugs test around 27 percent THC).

The Solar-Powered Farm
What: Emerald Pharms
Where: Hopland, California

What's the deal: The world's first solar-powered dispensary is on a picture-perfect, twelve-acre sustainable farm that calls itself a "permaculture oasis." Definitely eat your organic edible on the gorgeous outdoor deck overlooking lily ponds and breathtaking hills.

What to get: Raw peanut butter cacao truffles. They're organic and non-GMO—obviously.

The Secret Art Gallery
What: ShowGrow
Where: Los Angeles, California

What's the deal: A cool dispensary in downtown LA that doubles as an under-the-radar art gallery, with photo portraits of Snoop Dogg and stencils by the artist Jesus Hands (who infamously vandalized the Hollywood sign to say "Hollyweed" in 2017) up for sale. There are also murals by street artists on the walls, and a grow room where you can check out their in-house plants.

What to get: Cannabis corn-chips and a watercolor by Marilyn Manson.

The Celebrity Weed Emporium
What: Buds & Roses
Where: Los Angeles, California

What's the deal: Sitting on Ventura Boulevard amid organic juiceries and expensive nail salons, Buds & Roses is where Hollywood directors and other entertainment industry-types like to shop. The sleek emporium stocks rare, highly coveted strains like Tangie and LA Confidential, and offers VIP services like free valet parking.

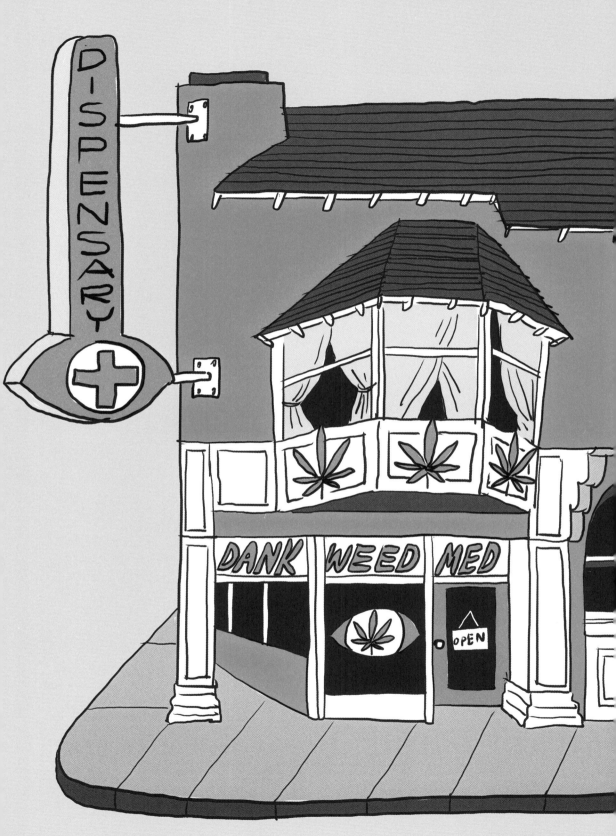

What to get: Flower from celebrity grower Kyle Kushman and indie movie director Kevin Smith.

The Hip Hotel Lobby
What: The Standard, Hollywood
Where: Los Angeles, California

What's the deal: A chic dispensary in the lobby of the Standard hotel stocks CBD lotions, gumdrops and other high-end treats, thanks to a partnership with celebrity favorite Lord Jones.

What to get: The limited-edition CBD gumdrops by rock band Sigur Rós, made with foraged Icelandic berries.

The Historic Fire Station
What: Cannabliss
Where: Eugene, Oregon

What's the deal: A long golden pole still runs through the red brick walls of this former fire station from 1913, thanks to Cannabliss's dedication to preserving the quirky charms of its unique locations—stop by the other location, too, in a former sorority house, and play a game of pool in the basement lounge.

What to get: Pop some caramel candy from Oregonian company Periodic Edibles to get a buzz on before you head over to the nearby Oregon Rail Heritage Center.

The Cannabis Museum
What: Dockside Cannabis
Where: Seattle, Washington

What's the deal: Dockside's Seattle shop packs a cute little museum full of cannabis apothecary jars and other historical stoner trinkets dating back to the 1800s.

What to get: Delicious concentrates that won awards at the 2017 Terpestival, which the dispensary also hosts.

The Smoothie Bar
What: Sea to Sky Alternative Healing Society
Where: Vancouver, Canada

What's the deal: A medical dispensary with a smoothie bar as well as an in-house naturopathic doctor.

What to get: Custom-blended, weed-infused juice.

The Medical Pioneers
What: Tikun Olam
Where: Tel Aviv, Israel

What's the deal: Tikun Olam means "repair the world" in Hebrew, and Tel Aviv's first and largest medical dispensary—which sits smack in the middle of the city—is leading the charge in cannabis research and normalizing cannabis use in Israel.

What to get: Medical-grade tinctures and capsules.

The Weed Vending Machine
What: BCPS Canada
Where: Vancouver, Canada

What's the deal: This Vancouver dispensary became an online sensation after it installed Canada's first weed vending machine in 2014. It's managed to fight off a city-ordered mandate to shut down and has even installed a second machine to keep up with demand.

What to get: Plastic balls containing dirt-cheap grams of weed from the gumball machine.

The *Portlandia* of Weed
What: Serra
Where: Portland, Oregon

What's the deal: Budtenders at this design-conscious store use origami-wrapped chopsticks to measure out your bud. There's an espresso machine on the white granite tabletop, and tons of super-stylish accessories like rose gold grinders, designer bongs, and combination-lock leather bags for hiding your stash.

What to get: Artisanal ceramic pipes and tiny glass bongs that double as home decor.

The Organic Oasis
What: Bloom City Club
Where: Ann Arbor, Michigan

What's the deal: This super-friendly and welcoming oasis is owned and run by women (one of its founders is nicknamed Ganjamama) and will immediately make you feel at home. The store specializes in organic, "craft" cannabis products from local sustainable growers—so you won't find any pesticides (or pesky men) here.

What to get: A nug of their small-batch cannabis flower.

The Walmart of Weed
What: Oasis Cannabis Superstore
Where: Denver, Colorado

What's the deal: This gigantic, fluorescent-lit weed supermarket stocks over 200 strains, 180 different pre-rolled joints, and an insane variety of bongs and pipes in row after row of glass display cases. If you're the type who likes to have way too many options, this is your one-stop shop.

What to get: Flower from local brands like Wanna, Lucky Edibles, Love's Oven, and Apothecanna. Thanks to high sales volumes, the strain menu changes frequently.

The Museum with a Jail Cell
What: Smokin Gun Apothecary
Where: Glendale, Colorado

What's the deal: This speakeasy-style "anti-prohibition museum" is open late and has an old-timey vibe: the bud counter is made from the wooden windows of an 1870s New Orleans bank, the walls are covered in artifacts from the Prohibition era, and there's a life-size replica of an old Mississippi jail cell in the back.

What to get: A "Prohibition Pass" (monthly membership) gets you cheap deals.

A Streetcar Named Weed
What: Discovery Bay Cannabis
Where: Port Townsend, Washington

What's the deal: A row of colorful old train cars in a quaint small town makes this the coziest dispensary in America.

What to get: Canna Vita chocolate, which comes in fun flavors like white chocolate raspberry and peanut butter and is perfect for making weed s'mores by the fire.

The Flashy Vegas Joint
What: Essence
Where: Las Vegas, Nevada

What's the deal: The first weed dispensary on Las Vegas's infamous Strip looks, very appropriately, like a gaudy, gargantuan nightclub: the 54,000-square-foot building's outer walls are covered in bright-green LED screens on all sides. Thankfully, the inside is way more chill—a sparsely furnished, gray-hued room stocking an amazing selection of premium-quality goods.

What to get: High-end weed lube (what happens in Vegas …).

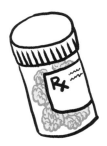

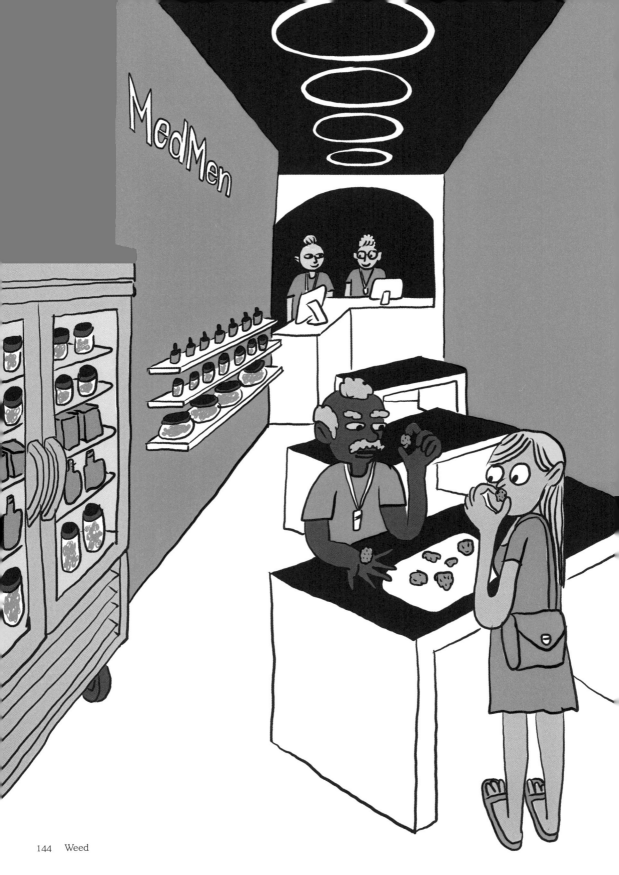

Dispensary Profile:
The Apple Store of Weed

What: MedMen
Where: Manhattan, New York City

What's the deal: This high-end cannabis chain's sleek NYC digs feel like the ubiquitous coffee chain had a baby with an Apple store.

MedMen's Manhattan flagship is nestled a stone's throw away from Bryant Park, smack in the middle of Fifth Avenue—a bourgie street lined with designer boutiques where Upper East Side socialites and soccer moms like to shop for handbags. Which is probably why, when it opened to much media fanfare in April 2018, it drew comparisons to the high-end department store Barney's.

MedMen is arguably the most well-known chain of dispensaries in America. The California-based company employs hundreds of people across several US states and Canada. Walk into one of its stores and you'll be greeted by smiling budtenders in identical company T-shirts, all clutching iPads.

Normalizing weed and bringing it into the mainstream is a huge part of MedMen's M.O. because—forget Barney's—one day they hope to become the go-to destination for casual users of pot. Opening a New York location in a pricey, high-traffic location is also part of that plan. The ten-thousand-square-foot Fifth Avenue shop really does look like an Apple Store, with futuristic

lighting, clean white walls, and budtenders running around in matching red T-shirts.

What to get: You can browse a range of vape pens, tinctures, and other cannabis products on the store's iPads. To streamline the often overwhelming experience of choosing what you want, everything is color-coded and classified according to mood: Wellness, Harmony, Awake, Calm, and Sleep. Even if you don't buy anything, you're still welcome to window shop (and drool) to your heart's content.

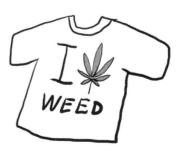

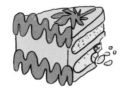

CAFÉS AND LOUNGES

Weed cafés offer an alternative vision of the future, one where socializing doesn't have to center entirely on alcohol. "Coffeeshops" have existed for decades in Amsterdam and aren't too different from regular bars—you pull up to the counter, flash some ID, and order weed from the menu. Then you pick a table to sit at and get stoned with your friends, assuaging your munchies with drinks and snacks.

Fancy weed lounges have also sprouted up in cities across the globe. These spots often charge membership fees, and in return you get access to everything from DJ parties to celebrity speakers, movie nights, and vape rentals.

More than anything, the best part about weed cafés and lounges is their sense of community and convenience. Contrary to popular opinion, weed can be a very social drug that you can enjoy in public. While there's nothing wrong with smoking in the comfort of your own home, sometimes you just want someone else to do all the work, sort out the playlist, and bring you food, too.

The Museum of Crazy Glass Pipes
What: Hitman
Where: Los Angeles, California

What's the deal: This custom-roasted coffee spot doubles as a members-only BYOC (bring your own cannabis) gathering space, with in-house dab rigs, an outdoor patio, and a collection of insane bongs displayed behind glass like museum pieces. A favorite among dudes who dab.

The Skater Hangout
What: HQ
Where: Barcelona, Spain

What's the deal: HQ stands for "Hempquarters," and this members-only spot is like a skater-hangout-meets-Soho-House for dabbers. It's got everything you've ever wanted from a weed social club: award-winning concentrates, sweet merch that looks like streetwear, weekend basketball tournaments, and DJ parties with pot pizza. It really doesn't get much cooler than this.

The Outdoor "Potio"
What: Hotbox Lounge and Café
Where: Toronto, Canada

What's the deal: Located in Toronto's busy Kensington Market, Hotbox is the oldest cannabis lounge in Canada. The front end of the room is a regular head shop selling pipes, papers, and

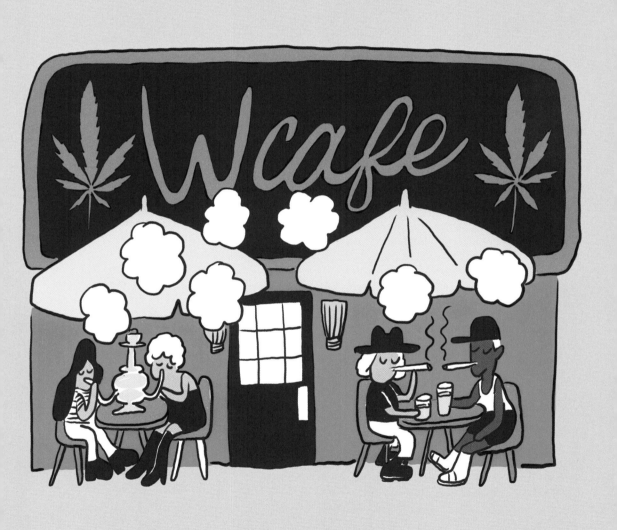

other accessories. But if you pay the $5 cover charge and bring your own weed, you can kick your feet up in the back area with drinks and snacks, and borrow a dab rig from the vape bar. Some advice: make a beeline for the giant, leafy outdoor patio and smoke your trees under the biggest umbrella.

The YMCA of Weed
What: Higher Limits
Where: Ontario, Canada

What's the deal: This sleek, modernist studio with brick walls and wood-paneled floors calls itself a cannabis community center. What that means: you can get your own locker to store your bongs and vapes, play video games on leather couches, order pizza from the restaurant downstairs, and attend talks by visiting celebrities—who have included one of Donald Trump's alleged mistresses, Stormy Daniels. (Seriously.)

The Celebrity Favorite
What: Green House Centrum
Where: Amsterdam, the Netherlands

What's the deal: This Hollywood favorite has been visited by Rihanna, Kid Cudi, and supermodel Cara Delevingne, and for good reason: it develops its own exclusive seeds using genetic science and has won more than forty Cannabis Cup awards. The owner, Arjan Roskam, was the star of VICE/HBO's 2011 documentary series Strain Hunters, adding even more cred to its celebrity appeal. The dimly lit space has an Old World vibe, with vintage maps covering the wood-paneled walls and tasseled lanterns hanging from the ceiling.

The Bohemian Crystal Garden
What: La Tertulia
Where: Amsterdam, the Netherlands

What's the deal: This sweet and cozy café has been run by a mother–daughter team

for over three decades and is frequented by older bohemians and artists. (Stars of the Real Housewives TV show have also been known to drop by.) It's located in one of Amsterdam's prettiest neighborhoods, and you can grab a seat on the terrace outside to gaze at the canal and the Van Gogh mural on the wall. Or head into the bright, airy, plant-filled interior and sit in the crystal garden full of healing stones like amethyst and quartz.

The Vegan Tarot Studio
What: Mumu to the Moon
Where: Amsterdam, the Netherlands

What's the deal: A combination vegan café and tarot studio serving dairy-free desserts and plant-based skincare lotions made from cold-pressed weed oils. Come for the oat milk latte, stay to get your tarot cards read.

The Cheers of Cannabis
What: Studio A64
Where: Colorado Springs, Colorado

What's the deal: This private club is so friendly that online reviewers call it the "Cheers of cannabis"—a place where every stoner knows your name. Tucked above a local bar, the women-owned space looks like your friend's stylish living room. Whether you're working on your laptop, jamming to a live band, or playing Canna-Bingo, don't forget to guzzle one of their infused smoothies.

America's First Weed Café
What: The Coffee Joint
Where: Denver, Colorado

What's the deal: The Coffee Joint became America's inaugural weed café in early 2018, when it received the first business permit for cannabis use from the city of Denver. The space also hosts yoga classes and crystal workshops, and if you ever run out of pot, just dip into their sister dispensary, 1136 Yuma, next door.

The Classy Sports Bar
What: Barbary Coast Dispensary
Where: San Francisco, California

What's the deal: Buy some weed at Barbary Coast Dispensary and you'll be granted access to their adjoining lounge, where chandeliers and tufted leather booths give it a strong resemblance to your dad's favorite steakhouse—complete with five HDTVs for watching the game.

The Dog-Friendly Sun Deck
What: NW Cannabis Club
Where: Portland, Oregon

What's the deal: Housed in a former strip club, this members-only hangout has a huge outdoor patio and shady gazebo perfect for smoking up with your furry friends at your feet. (You could even give them some CBD pet tincture.) When the sun sets, take a seat at the fifty-foot dab bar inside for one of their nightly events—which include burlesque shows and stoned karaoke—or go down to the basement lounge to try your hand at the pool table.

The Firelit Lounge with a Farmers Market
What: Planet Paradise
Where: Toronto, Canada

What's the deal: This dimly lit lounge has an extra-cozy vibe thanks to its multiple fireplaces and the kitschy art lining the walls. The bar serves everything from cereal to organic fruit juices, and if you're lucky you might even walk into the weekly Cannabis Farmers Market, where you can stock up on the best local flowers and edibles.

The Swanky Musician's Salon
What: Joe's Smokers Club Marbella
Where: Marbella, Spain

What's the deal: This sleek, members-only lounge looks like a hip hotel lobby and comes with a simple policy: "No nuns, no children, and no non-smokers." Taking a seat on the zebra-print sofa to

strum one of the many musical instruments lying around while smoking all-organic weed, you might feel like you're jamming in a rock star's penthouse.

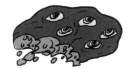

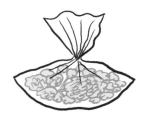

DRIVE-THROUGHS

There's a particular kind of lazy satisfaction that comes from being given what you're craving without having to get off your butt. Nothing quite beats rolling up to a drive-through in your car, sticking out your hand, and receiving a paper bag with a delicious burger inside. Or, even better: a joint.

Weed drive-throughs. We can all agree that this was inevitable. Yet it's a pretty recent phenomenon: the first one only popped up in 2017, in Colorado. Since then, several others have opened across the US, and there's no doubt that many more will join them soon.

Unlike, say, a McDonald's, you can't actually just pull up to a window and start barking your order into a static-y intercom. Since weed drive-throughs are subject to the same laws as dispensaries, everyone in the car will first need to get their ID checked, even if you're in the back seat. A lot of them are also cash-only, so don't forget to bring some dough. But yes, just like a fast-food chain,

there will probably be a menu board that you'll be tempted to order everything from, and a pick-up window where a staffer will hand you a bag of treats with a smile. Just remember not to get (too) stoned if you're driving, because if a cop pulls you over, you could get slapped with a cannabis DUI, which are on the rise.

While they might sound like a fun and somewhat outlandish novelty, weed drive-throughs actually have a more practical purpose than you might expect: serving the elderly and disabled, as well as medical patients who might be in too much pain to get out of their car. The elderly are a rapidly growing market in the cannabis world, so don't be surprised if you see a couple of grandmas driving very slowly in line in front of you.

Often open late or 24-hours, and able to serve you within minutes, the amazing convenience of weed drive-throughs is ultimately what guarantees that they will soon be lining streets all over the world. Now if only you could get fries with that.

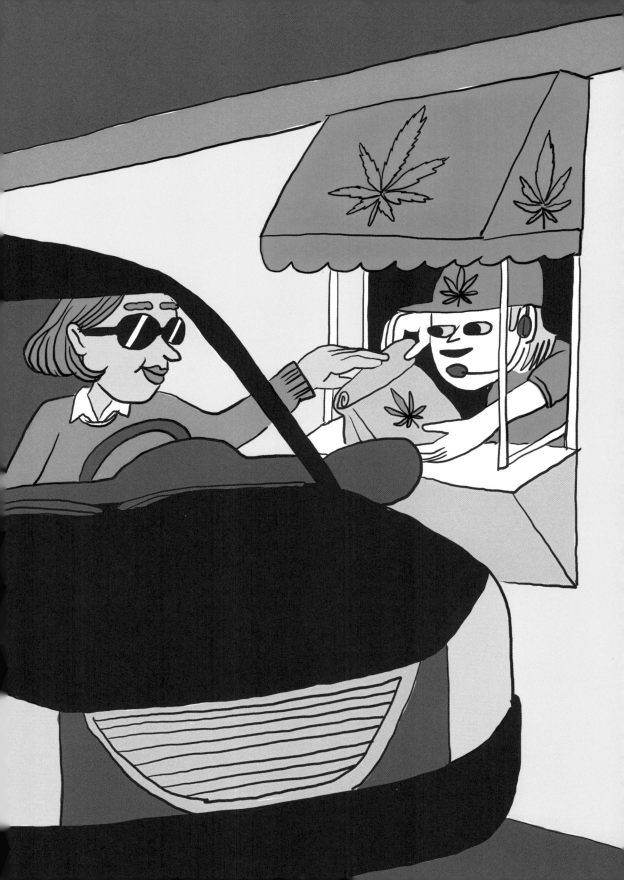

What: The Tumbleweed Express
Where: Parachute, Colorado

What's the deal: A car-wash garage in a tiny town where you'll find the world's first weed drive-through.

Parachute in Colorado has a population of just 1,100 people. Dark, jagged silhouettes of mountains surround the tiny area, which, like many other towns that line America's highways, doesn't have much to offer visitors beyond liquor stores, fast-food chains, and gas stations. Until a few years ago, you'd probably have driven right past if you were on a road trip, maybe stopping for a few minutes to grab a snack and to pee. It definitely wasn't the kind of place you'd expect to become the go-to weed destination for drivers passing along Interstate 70.

In 2014, when legalization hit Colorado, Parachute initially recoiled at the thought of stoner tourists descending on the town and decided to ban all cannabis businesses. But the area desperately needed money. A big part of its local economy depended on natural gas, and a recent slump in the gas industry was costing Parachute a third of its sales tax revenue.

Locals realized that if they essentially replaced gas with weed as their main economy, they could make bank. Some 135,000 visitors stop by Parachute's popular rest area every year, and chances were that a lot of people in those cars were probably down to get stoned. Parachute was also in a prime position to reap the rewards of the Green Rush—the two towns next to it, Grand Junction to the west and Rifle to the east, had similarly outlawed recreational weed. So in June 2015, in a somewhat controversial vote, the locals voted to lift the ban.

The first Tumbleweed dispensary in Parachute opened in February 2016 at the edge of town. It's a huge, handsome store with three giant green medical cross signs hanging outside, and a mountain-lodge-meets-country-saloon vibe once you step in. Everything from the walls to the counters is made from reclaimed wood, and products are displayed under elegant steel lamps in a row of wooden barrels resting on their sides behind the bar.

Tumbleweed's owner, fifty-eight-year-old businessman Mark Smith, is a pretty enterprising dude. He started out as a pawnshop magnate and sold the twenty-three stores he owned to jump into the cannabis business in Colorado when he smelled a dank opportunity. One night, while working alone in the dispensary, he noticed that the car wash across the street had a "for sale" sign. That gave him an idea: so many people were coming by the dispensary after-hours, when it had already closed. Rather than turn away business, why not open a drive-through window that would stay open late? "I didn't have some big epiphany," he told the local press, "I just saw a need for our customers."

Smith immediately bought the car wash. He decided to keep the building's existing infra-structure, which means you can't actually just drive up to a window from the street to pick up your weed. Instead, you pull up, stopping to check out the signboard—which looks a lot like the ones you see at fast-food drive-throughs, but with weed on the menu. The gate swings open so you can drive into the dark-brown garage, which is lit with bright fluorescent lights. As the gate closes behind you, you see a friendly face with an earpiece poking out of a wooden booth on your left, ready to take your order.

When Smith opened the Tumbleweed in 2017 on April 20 (when else?), the media understandably freaked out. After all, no one had thought of this brilliant idea before, which in retrospect seems so obvious. Tumbleweed inadvertently kicked off a new trend; several other weed drive-throughs have since opened across the country. These days, Parachute, which Smith says is now "very supportive," makes 30 percent of its revenue from cannabis sales. There are now seven dispensaries in the town—that's one for every 170 people.

The Native American-Owned
What: NuWu Cannabis Marketplace
Where: Las Vegas, Nevada

What's the deal: A weed supermarket owned by a Native American tribe in the heart of Sin City.

When NuWu opened its doors in Las Vegas in October 2017, some two hundred tribal leaders and families from across Nevada celebrated with a party that featured traditional Native American songs, chants, and dances.

The 15,500-square-foot dispensary was a big achievement for the Southern Paiute tribe, which has just fifty-six members ("Nuwu" means "Southern Paiute people"). It is Nevada's largest cannabis retail facility, and the first on tribal land. Since Native American tribes are exempt from taxes according to federal law, weed could be a huge financial boon for these communities. "We just wanted to be able to play with the big dogs up here," Paiute Tribe Chairman Benny Tso, a broad-shouldered man with thick black glasses and tattoos on both of his beefy forearms, told the *Las Vegas Sun*.

You can find NuWu's drive-through by pulling up along the side of the dispensary. The booth, which juts out from the warehouse's outer wall, is actually a converted bank vault window with bulletproof glass. You can choose from a limited menu of the dispensary's most popular items, or, if you order online, pick from the full range of seven hundred items. The window is also open 24 hours a day, so you can easily pop in and out—especially since they aim to serve you in less than a minute after you place your order.

The Munchie Paradise
What: All Greens
Where: Sun City, Arizona

What's the deal: A medical dispensary in a former bank, with amazing edibles.

All Greens took over a former bank with an already operating drive-through for its ATMs, so it simply swapped the cash machines for weed and changed the fluorescent lights to a clubby neon green. The Arizona dispensary, which has been running since 2013, is medical-only—although there's a clinic right there, so you can get your medical card when you arrive. How convenient.

You'll also need to register inside the dispensary and go through two security checks before you can use the drive-through, which is a bit of a pain but worth it. All Greens claims to have the largest variety of edibles in the state, including marshmallow crispy squares, organic peanut butter, and vegan chocolate cookies. Plus, it has its own grow facility, so you know you're getting top-notch products.

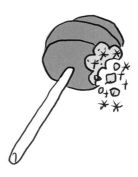

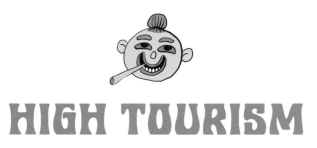

HIGH TOURISM

As legal weed sweeps across certain lucky corners of the world, some entrepreneurial spirits have seized the opportunity to cater to the influx of tourists flocking to these areas.

In California's Coachella Valley, for example, so many new grow facilities and dispensaries have sprung up that the region is jokingly referred to as "Tokechella." Many of the hot spring hotels that have been serving Hollywood starlets and mobsters for decades have now turned into cannabis-friendly resorts where you're allowed to smoke while you roam around the property or sit by the pool. On the other hand, in other countries, like Uruguay, museums are being erected to preserve weed history, educate the public, and dispel lingering stigma.

From weed party buses to wellness retreats, these are some of the best vacations a pothead could ask for.

The Bud-and-Breakfast
What: Hicksville Pines Bud & Breakfast
Where: Idyllwild, California

What's the deal: This weed-friendly bed-and-breakfast lets you get stoned in all of its common areas, which also means you have to be twenty-one or over to stay here. Each of the delightfully decorated rooms has a different theme, like "Dolly Parton" or "Haunted Mansion," but obviously you know where you're staying: Room 420. It's the only room with an en-suite vaporizer.

The Only Weed Museum in South America
What: Museo del Cannabis
Where: Montevideo, Uruguay

What's the deal: Uruguay legalized weed in 2013, and locals can now buy herb at their neighborhood pharmacy. This museum, which got some of its collection from Amsterdam's Hash, Marihuana & Hemp Museum, features an array of artifacts in glass displays that delve into the variety of uses for the plant, from food to clothing and medicine.

The Weed Party Bus
What: West Coast Cannabis Tours
Where: San Diego, California

What's the deal: A party bus that lets you smoke on board, feeds you beer and cannabis trivia, then takes you to a dispensary, a bong-making demo, and an edibles cooking class—all in an afternoon. Who says stoners don't get shit done?

The Women's Cannabis Retreat
What: Ganja Goddess Getaways
Where: Southern California

What's the deal: A series of weekend retreats around Southern California where only women are allowed. There are art classes, stand-up comedy acts, educational talks about how cannabis can impact women's health and sexuality … and of course, lots and lots of yoga.

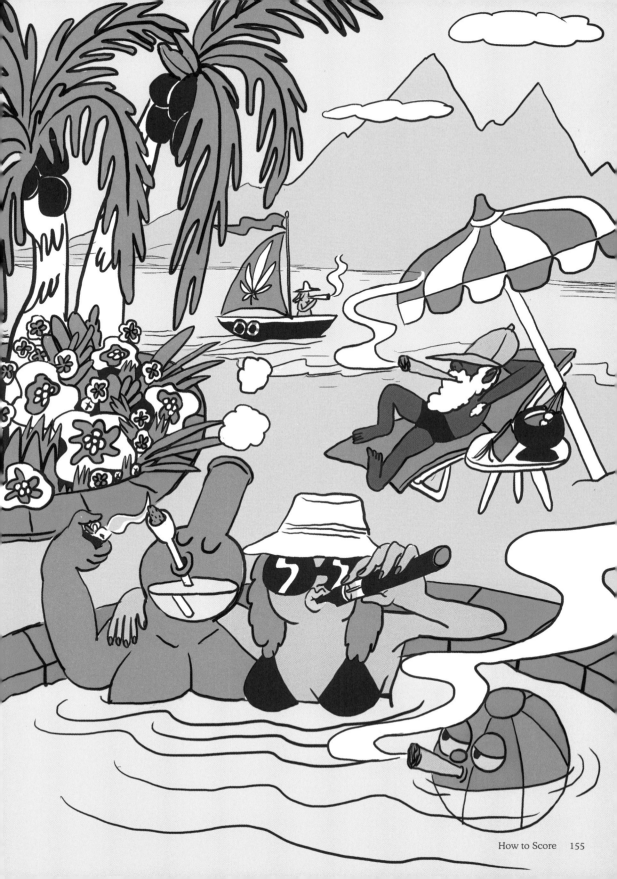

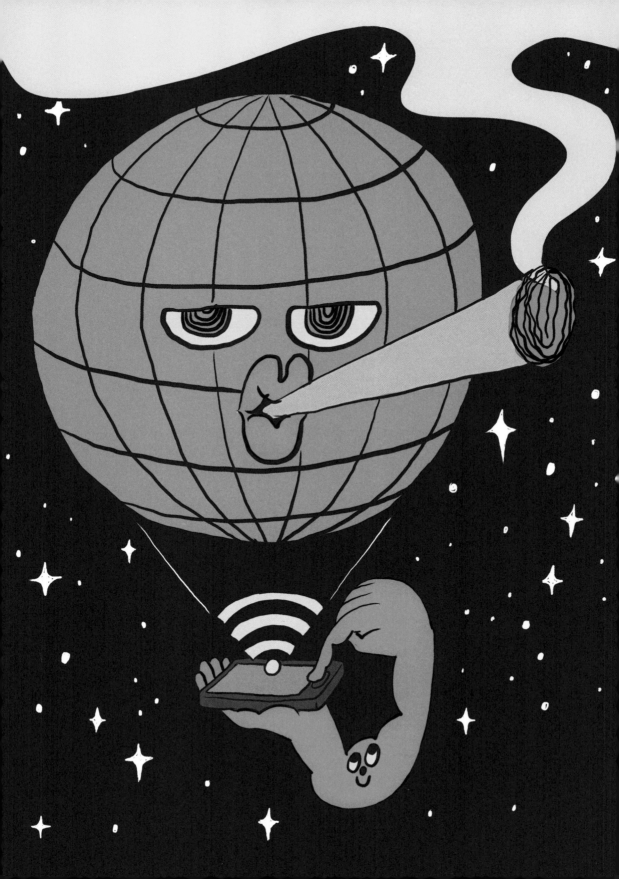

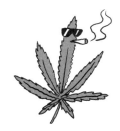

WORLD WIDE WEED

These days you can do everything online, so here's an index of websites where you can find useful weed reviews, buy cool accessories, order home delivery, and so much more.

Leafly (leafly.com)
A detailed index of thousands of cannabis strains, with information on their chemical compounds, effects, and flavor profiles, and crowd-sourced reviews.

A Proper High (aproperhigh.com)
Entertaining reviews of products ranging from edibles to flowers, written by cannabis insiders and with a focus on specific weed brands rather than strains.

Eaze (eaze.com)
A California-based weed home-delivery service that will pick up from local dispensaries and deliver your order straight to your door, usually within twenty minutes, and with cute packaging to boot.

Weed Maps (weedmaps.com)
Like Yelp, but for finding the best dispensaries, doctors, and delivery services near you.

Mister Green (green-mister.com)
A cool, California-based online store hawking T-shirts, tote bags, ashtrays, and other accessories that look more Silver Lake hipster than tie-dye hippie (thank god).

Broccoli (broccolimag.com)
Founded by Kinfolk's former creative director, this feminist weed magazine combines artistic visual spreads with well-written feature stories on cultural topics that go beyond just cannabis (see p. 124).

DankGals (dankgals.com)
This online shop is run by Asian American stoners and sells some of the cutest glasswear and accessories on the market, including a Sriracha bottle-shaped dab rig and pipes carved out of crystals.

Merry Jane (merryjane.com)
Snoop Dogg's media company is hoping to be the VICE of weed, with a combination of in-depth journalism, videos, and entertaining essays.

High Times (hightimes.com)
The oldest and most respected weed magazine in the game.

Herb (herb.co)
A weed blog that specializes in breaking news from around the world, useful tips, and edibles recipes.

The Stoner Mom (thestonermom.com)
This site provides tips, reviews, recipes, and podcasts for moms who smoke weed.

The Cannabist (thecannabist.co)
A weed website chock full of news, reviews, and stories about weed culture.

AUTHOR BIOS

Michelle Lhooq is a music and weed journalist in Los Angeles who writes about sex (especially queer culture and feminism), drugs (…obviously), and crazy raves. She was born in Singapore and has lived in Tokyo, upstate New York, Paris, Shanghai, and Beijing. In 2007 she moved to New York City to study comparative literature at Columbia University. She was a music editor at *VICE* in Brooklyn for many years, reporting on the wildest and weirdest parties around the world. In 2017 she moved to California to witness the weed revolution—and ended up writing this book. She currently contributes to the *Los Angeles Times*, *New York Magazine*, *FADER*, *Teen Vogue*, and *Pitchfork*, among other publications. You can admire her perfectly rolled joints at @michellelhooq.

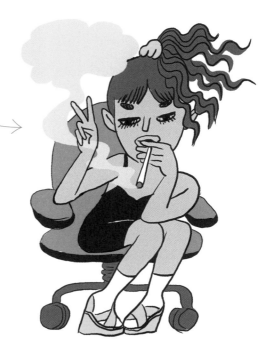

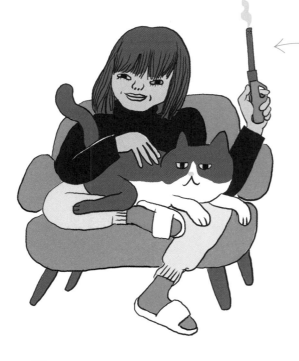

Thu Tran is an artist and performer who makes comics, videos, and video games. She smoked socially in her twenties, became a daily wake-and-baker in her thirties, and lately just eats cold pats of weed butter every now and again. She created and hosted stoner cooking shows for IFC (*Food Party*) and MTV (*Late Night Munchies*) and has made short-form videos for Adult Swim, Super Deluxe, and other outlets. Her video games and video installations have been shown at the Museum of the Moving Image and Babycastles in New York City, Fantastic Arcade in Austin, and at various art spaces, educational institutions, and events around the world. Her comics have been published by Peow Studio and Kuš Komiks. She conducts her business from NYC and spends most of her time in her studio in her hometown of Cleveland with her voluptuous tuxedo cat, Silk.

ACKNOWLEDGMENTS

Michelle Lhooq: I am so stoked that my first book is about weed—and for that, I am forever grateful to my editor, Ali Gitlow, and the team at Prestel. Ali, thank you for believing in me and guiding me through this eye-opening journey with infinite patience and support. I am going to miss our long-distance Skype calls. Thu, during my darkest moments of self-doubt, your brilliant work was my beacon of hope. You're a genius weirdo, and the reason why this book is *so cute*. To all the women and people of color who let me interview them, and to those behind the scenes who helped: you're the best! Kudos to all my weed journalist friends, especially Lindsay for taking me to parties—they gave me so much material (and free swag). Thanks to my family, for putting up with me.

Most of all, this one goes out to all the stoners who've picked up this book. I hope you wander around this world with joints forever hanging from your lips.

Thu Tran: I am thankful to have had a valid, professional excuse to draw weed leaves all day. Thank you to our editor, Ali Gitlow, for making this book happen, for bringing us all together, for trusting me to do this, and for your thoughtful direction throughout this project. To Michelle Lhooq, for writing this book, which has been a joy to read, informative, and relatable. Thanks to Nick Shea, our designer, for laying out this book and making it look as nice as it does. To my parents, for their boundless love and support: I hope you never see this book! To my brother Tuan, for making the dankest sticks of weed butter. They got me through some of the longer days of drawing; your product is very potent. I am appreciative of Vinald Francis for smoking me up for the first time during a lunch break in design class back in college. Thank you for making my first experience so friendly, for changing my life forever, and for the recent long talks. You are a great friend. To all the drug dealers and weed delivery people, I am grateful for your service, your kind nugs, and the chill conversations. Lastly, thanks to weed itself, for being a reliable enabler of relaxation and laffs.

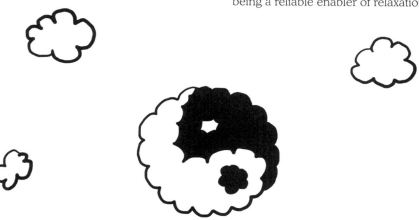